Functional and Cosmetic Eyelid Surgery

Editor

GREGORY H. BRANHAM

FACIAL PLASTIC SURGERY CLINICS OF NORTH AMERICA

www.facialplastic.theclinics.com

Consulting Editor
J. REGAN THOMAS

May 2016 • Volume 24 • Number 2

ELSEVIER

1600 John F. Kennedy Boulevard • Suite 1800 • Philadelphia, Pennsylvania, 19103-2899

http://www.theclinics.com

FACIAL PLASTIC SURGERY CLINICS OF NORTH AMERICA Volume 24, Number 2
May 2016 ISSN 1064-7406, ISBN-13: 978-0-323-44463-7

Editor: Jessica McCool
Developmental Editor: Alison Swety

Facial Plastic Surgery Clinics of North America (ISSN 1064-7406) is published quarterly by Elsevier Inc., 360 Park Avenue South, New York, NY 10010-1710. Months of issue are February, May, August, and November. Business and Editorial Offices: 1600 John F. Kennedy Blvd., Suite 1800, Philadelphia, PA 19103-2899. Periodicals postage paid at New York, NY, and additional mailing offices. Subscription prices are $390.00 per year (US individuals), $575.00 per year (US institutions), $445.00 per year (Canadian individuals), $716.00 per year (Canadian institutions), $535.00 per year (foreign individuals), $716.00 per year (foreign institutions), $100.00 per year (US students), and $255.00 per year (foreign students). Foreign air speed delivery is included in all *Clinics* subscription prices. All prices are subject to change without notice. POSTMASTER: Send address changes to *Facial Plastic Surgery Clinics*, Elsevier Health Sciences Division, Subscription Customer Service, 3251 Riverport Lane, Maryland Heights, MO 63043. **Customer service: 1-800-654-2452 (US and Canada); 1-314-447-8871 (outside US and Canada); Fax: 314-447-8029; E-mail: journalscustomerservice-usa@elsevier.com (for print support); journalsonline support-usa@elsevier.com (for online support).**

Reprints. For copies of 100 or more of articles in this publication, please contact the Commercial Reprints Department, Elsevier Inc., 360 Park Avenue South, New York, NY 10010-1710. Tel.: 212-633-3874; Fax: 212-633-3820; E-mail: reprints@elsevier.com.

Facial Plastic Surgery Clinics of North America is covered in *MEDLINE/PubMed* (*Index Medicus*).

Contributors

CONSULTING EDITOR

J. REGAN THOMAS, MD, FACS
Professor and Chairman, Department of
Otolaryngology, University of Illinois at
Chicago, Chicago, Illinois

EDITOR

GREGORY H. BRANHAM, MD
Professor and Chief, Facial Plastic and
Reconstructive Surgery, Department of
Otolaryngology–Head and Neck Surgery,
Washington University School of Medicine,
Washington University in St Louis, St Louis;
Facial Plastic Surgery Center, Creve Coeur,
Missouri

AUTHORS

GREGORY H. BRANHAM, MD
Professor and Chief, Facial Plastic and
Reconstructive Surgery, Department of
Otolaryngology–Head and Neck Surgery,
Washington University School of
Medicine, Washington University in
St Louis, St Louis; Facial Plastic
Surgery Center, Creve Coeur,
Missouri

JOHN J. CHI, MD
Assistant Professor, Division of Facial
Plastic and Reconstructive Surgery,
Washington University School of Medicine,
Washington University in St Louis,
St Louis; Facial Plastic Surgery Center,
Creve Coeur, Missouri

STEVEN M. COUCH, MD, FACS
Assistant Professor, Oculofacial Plastic and
Reconstructive Surgery, Department of
Ophthalmology and Visual Sciences,
Washington University School of Medicine,
Washington University in St Louis, St Louis,
Missouri

SHAUN C. DESAI, MD
Assistant Professor, Division of Facial Plastic
and Reconstructive Surgery, Department of
Otolaryngology–Head and Neck Surgery,
Johns Hopkins University School of Medicine,
Baltimore; Bethesda, Maryland

GABRIELA MABEL ESPINOZA, MD
Clinical Associate Professor, Department of
Ophthalmology, Saint Louis University Eye
Institute, Saint Louis University School of
Medicine, St Louis, Missouri

DEE ANNA GLASER, MD
Interim Chair and Professor; Director,
Division of Cosmetic and Laser Surgery;
Department of Dermatology, Saint Louis
University School of Medicine, St Louis,
Missouri

SAMUEL HAHN, MD
Clinical Fellow, Facial Plastic and
Reconstructive Surgery, Department of
Otolaryngology–Head and Neck Surgery,
Washington University School of Medicine,
Washington University in St Louis, St Louis,
Missouri

MORRIS E. HARTSTEIN, MD, FACS
Director, Ophthalmic Plastic Surgery;
Department of Ophthalmology, Assaf
Harofeh Medical Center, Tel Aviv University
Sackler School of Medicine, Raanana,
Israel

JOHN B. HOLDS, MD, FACS
Clinical Professor, Departments of
Ophthalmology and Otolaryngology–Head and
Neck Surgery, Saint Louis University School of
Medicine, St Louis, Missouri; Ophthalmic
Plastic and Cosmetic Surgery, Inc, Des Peres,
Missouri

KAVEH KARIMNEJAD, MD
Department of Otolaryngology–Head and Neck
Surgery, Saint Louis University School of
Medicine, St Louis, Missouri

ANASTASIA KURTA, DO
Department of Dermatology, Saint Louis
University School of Medicine, St Louis,
Missouri

MICHAEL G. NEIMKIN, MD
Ophthalmic Plastic and Cosmetic Surgery
Inc; Instructor, Department of Ophthalmology
and Visual Sciences, Washington University
School of Medicine, Washington University in
St Louis, St Louis, Missouri

ANGELA MICHELLE PROST, FNP-BC
Department of Ophthalmology, Saint Louis
University Eye Institute, Saint Louis University
School of Medicine, St Louis, Missouri

JORDAN P. SAND, MD
Resident, Department of Otolaryngology–Head
and Neck Surgery, Washington University
School of Medicine, Washington University in
St Louis, St Louis, Missouri

SCOTT WALEN, MD, FRCS(C)
Assistant Professor, Department of
Otolaryngology–Head and Neck Surgery,
Saint Louis University School of Medicine,
St Louis, Missouri

BOVEY Z. ZHU, MD
Resident, Department of Otolaryngology–Head
and Neck Surgery, Walter Reed National
Military Medical Center, Bethesda, Maryland

Contents

Slight alterations in the intricate anatomy of the upper and lower eyelid or their underlying structures can have pronounced consequences for ocular esthetics and function. The understanding of periorbital structures and their interrelationships continues to evolve and requires consideration when performing complex eyelid interventions. Maintaining a detailed appreciation of this region is critical to successful cosmetic or reconstructive surgery. This article presents a current review of the anatomy of the upper and lower eyelid with a focus on surgical implications.

The eyes and periocular area are the central aesthetic unit of the face. Facial aging is a dynamic process that involves skin, subcutaneous soft tissues, and bony structures. An understanding of what is perceived as youthful and beautiful is critical for success. Knowledge of the functional aspects of the eyelid and periocular area can identify pre-preoperative red flags.

Periorbital rejuvenation requires a careful understanding of the interplay between the eyelids, brow, forehead, and midface. Reversing periorbital signs of aging requires a correction of volume loss, soft tissue ptosis, and skin changes. Many surgical and nonsurgical techniques exist to treat the aging periorbital region; however, careful consideration of the patient's complaints and existing anatomy is critical to achieving a safe and esthetically pleasing outcome.

Upper lid blepharoplasty is a common procedure for restoration and rejuvenation of the upper eyelids that can be performed safely and reliably. Understanding the anatomy and aging process of the brow–upper lid aesthetic unit along with properly assessing the excesses and deficiencies of the periorbital region helps to formulate an appropriate surgical plan. Volume deficiency in the aging upper lid may require corrective augmentation. Preexisting asymmetries and ptosis need to be identified and discussed before surgery. Standardized photography along with a candid discussion regarding patients' desired outcomes and realistic expectations are essential to a successful outcome.

cornea. Defects of the upper eyelid may be due to congenital defects or traumatic injury or follow oncologic resection. This article focuses on reconstruction due to loss of tissue. Multiple surgeries may be needed to reach the desired results, addressing loss of tissue and then loss of function. Each defect is unique and the laxity and availability of surrounding tissue vary. Knowing the most common techniques for repair assists surgeons in the multifaceted planning that takes place.

Lower eyelid defects are common, and a systematic approach to reconstruction of the lower eyelid is required. Attention to the bilaminar eyelid anatomy and canthal support structures, with efforts to maintain functionally important structures, such as the lacrimal canalicular system, is vital to appropriate lower eyelid reconstruction. Techniques of advancement and rotation flaps and grafting of skin and mucosa are mainstays of lower eyelid reconstruction. An appropriate armamentarium of techniques allows for optimal surgical results.

Eyelid surgery consists of challenging reconstructive and cosmetic procedures. Because of the complex anatomy and corresponding vital functions of the upper and lower eyelids, the avoidance of eyelid complications is of vital importance. Complications after eyelid surgery include basic complications (infection, granuloma) and vision-threatening complications. Preoperative history, physical examination, surgical planning, and meticulous surgical technique must be undertaken to prevent complications after eyelid surgery. In addition, patient knowledge, expectations, and motivations must be determined before surgery is performed.

FACIAL PLASTIC SURGERY CLINICS OF NORTH AMERICA

RELATED INTEREST

Clinics in Plastic Surgery, January 2015 (Vol. 42, No. 1)
Lower Lid and Face: Multispecialty Approach
Babak Azizzadeh and Guy G. Massry, *Editors*
http://www.plasticsurgery.theclinics.com/

THE CLINICS ARE AVAILABLE ONLINE!
Access your subscription at:
www.theclinics.com

Preface
Functional and Cosmetic Eyelid Surgery

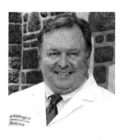

Gregory H. Branham, MD
Editor

I am excited to present this issue solely devoted to the upper and lower eyelids and surrounding periorbital tissues. Rather than addressing only cosmetic procedures, we wanted to address the periorbital region from both a reconstructive and an esthetic approach. It is my firm belief that each of these approaches to the periorbital region enhances the knowledge and skill of the periorbital surgeon.

While the title conveys a concentration on the eyelids, the editor and each contributor understand and convey a comprehensive approach to the periorbital region. In the past, eyelid surgery was viewed as isolated procedures performed alone or in conjunction with other aging facial procedures. State-of-the-art rejuvenation of the periorbital region focuses on restoring the natural youthful contours of the region through a combination of surgical and nonsurgical techniques.

Reconstruction of the upper and lower eyelids is essential to maintain function and preserve vision, and many of the principles utilized in reconstructive procedures apply to the esthetic restoration of the periorbital region. There is no doubt that

the esthetic surgeon is made better by the use of these reconstructive tools and vice versa.

I would like to thank all of the contributors who worked diligently to provide the latest information on this subject. It is an honor and privilege to call them colleagues. They represent the best and most experienced in this field and have labored to provide their expertise to you in this issue. I have learned much from each of them and commend their knowledge to you.

Gregory H. Branham, MD
Facial Plastic and Reconstructive Surgery
Department of Otolaryngology–Head
and Neck Surgery
Washington University in St Louis
Facial Plastic Surgery Center
1020 North Mason Road, Suite 205
Creve Coeur, MO 63141, USA

E-mail address:
branhamg@wustl.edu
Website:
http://facialplasticsurgery.wustl.edu

Facial Plast Surg Clin N Am 24 (2016) ix
http://dx.doi.org/10.1016/j.fsc.2016.02.001
1064-7406/16/$ – see front matter © 2016 Published by Elsevier Inc.

Surgical Anatomy of the Eyelids

Jordan P. Sand, MD[a], Bovey Z. Zhu, MD[b], Shaun C. Desai, MD[c],*

KEYWORDS

- Upper eyelid • Lower eyelid • Blepharoplasty • Orbicularis oculi • Orbital septum • Anatomy

KEY POINTS

- The complex anatomy of the upper and lower eyelid and its interrelation with underlying structures has important consequences for both esthetics and function.
- A strict understanding of the anatomic relationships of the eyelid components will help the facial plastic surgeon approach eyelid surgery safely and effectively.
- The structures of the upper and lower lid have many contiguous structures but several key differences that are important to recognize when performing periorbital procedures.

INTRODUCTION

The surgical anatomy of the eyelid is one of the most complex in the head and neck, and a thorough understanding of the intricacies is paramount for facial plastic surgeons. The eyelid functions to provide lubrication to the cornea while also serving as a barrier to foreign bodies. Lubrication of the corneal surface is achieved by a protective tear film, which is spread over the surface by periodic blinking. A multilayered tear film is formed from the lacrimal gland as well as small glands in the eyelid. The combination of mucus, oil, and aqueous materials provides a lubricating film that is eventually broken down by the atmosphere. Periodic blinking helps to replenish the balance of this important tear film.[1]

The normal adult eyelids form an elliptical palpebral fissure measuring 8 to 11 mm vertically at the pupillary meridian by 27 to 30 mm horizontally.[2] There are subtle but important differences when evaluating the upper and lower eyelid. The upper lid rests 1 to 2 mm below the superior limbus of the iris, while the lower lid rests along the inferior limbus.[2] The lateral canthus is 2 to 4 mm higher than the medial canthus, and the interpalpebral distance is 10 to 12 mm[1] (**Fig. 1**).

The upper and lower eyelids are composed of several analogous structures. Most commonly, these structures can be divided into an anterior, middle, and posterior lamellae. The anterior lamella refers to the skin and orbicularis oculi muscle of the eyelid. The posterior lamella refers to the retractors, superior or inferior tarsal muscle, tarsus, and the conjunctiva. Some investigators also reference the orbital septum as the middle lamella; however, this can vary depending on the source. The through-and-through layers are different depending on one's vertical position over the eyelid and are discussed in the following sections (**Fig. 2**).

ANTERIOR LAMELLAE
Upper Eyelid

The skin is the most superficial layer of the upper eyelid and is unique in that it is the thinnest skin of the body. The necessity for rapid eyelid

Disclosure Statement: The authors have nothing to disclose.
[a] Department of Otolaryngology–Head and Neck Surgery, Washington University School of Medicine, 660 South Euclid Avenue, Campus Box 8115, St Louis, MO 63110, USA; [b] Department of Otolaryngology–Head and Neck Surgery, Walter Reed National Military Medical Center, 8901 Wisconsin Avenue, Bethesda, MD 20889, USA; [c] Division of Facial Plastic and Reconstructive Surgery, Department of Otolaryngology–Head & Neck Surgery, Johns Hopkins University School of Medicine, 6420 Rockledge Drive, Suite 4920, Bethesda, MD 20817, USA
* Corresponding author. 6420 Rockledge Drive, Suite 4920, Bethesda, MD 20817.
E-mail address: sdesai27@jhmi.edu

Facial Plast Surg Clin N Am 24 (2016) 89–95
http://dx.doi.org/10.1016/j.fsc.2015.12.001

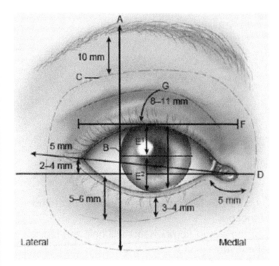

Fig. 1. Topography of the eyelid. (A) The highest point of the brow is at, or lateral to, the lateral limbus. (B) The inferior edge of the brow is shown 10 mm superior to the supraorbital rim. (C) Also shown are ranges for average palpebral height (10–12 mm), width (28–30 mm) (D), and upper lid fold (8–11 mm, with gender and racial differences). Note that the lateral canthus is 2 to 4 mm higher than the medial canthus. (E) Intrapalpebral distance measures 10 to 12 mm. E1, mean reflex distance 1; E2, mean reflex distance 2. (F) Palpebral width. (G) Upper lid fold is 8 to 11 mm. (*From* Most SP, Mobley SR, Larrabee WF Jr. Anatomy of the eyelids. [review]. Facial Plast Surg Clin North Am 2005;13:488; with permission.)

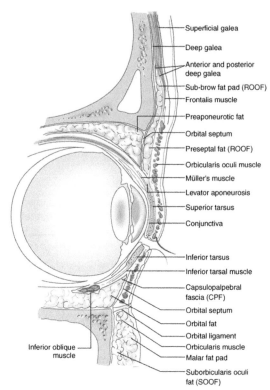

Fig. 2. Cross-sectional anatomy of the upper and lower lids. The capsulopalpebral fascia and inferior tarsal muscle are retractors of the lower lid, whereas Müller muscle, the levator muscle, and its aponeurosis are retractors of the upper lid. Note the preseptal positioning of the ROOF and suborbicularis oculi fat. The orbitomalar ligament arises from the arcus marginalis of the inferior orbital rim and inserts on the skin of the lower lid, forming the nasojugal fold. (*From* Most SP, Mobley SR, Larrabee WF Jr. Anatomy of the eyelids. [review]. Facial Plast Surg Clin North Am 2005;13:489; with permission.)

movements during blinking requires the skin to be highly flexible. Because of this intrinsic quality, there are very few adnexal structures or sebaceous glands in this skin. From a reconstruction standpoint, this often poses a challenge, as the reconstructive dictum of "replacing like with like" limits options to using the contralateral eyelid skin as the ideal source. Other skin graft donor sites can be too thick and may become cosmetically unacceptable.

Just below the skin of the upper eyelid lies the orbicularis oculi (**Fig. 3**). The orbicularis oculi is divided into orbital and palpebral portions. The orbital portion is formed by concentric muscle fibers arising from the medial canthal tendon, and it functions to close the eyes tightly. Laterally, the fibers insert subcutaneously and contribute to the formation of "crow's feet."[3] The palpebral portion consists of semilunar muscle fibers that span the medial and lateral canthal tendons. It can be further subdivided into pretarsal and preseptal portions, named by the structures they overlie. Medially, each subdivision arises from 2 heads, with the superficial heads arising from the insertion of the medial canthal tendon onto the

anterior lacrimal crest, while the deep heads insert near the posterior lacrimal crest.[4] The medial portions of the palpebral orbicularis help with the lacrimal apparatus.[5] Laterally, the fibers condense to form the lateral canthal tendon, which inserts onto Whitnall tubercle, located approximately 4 mm posterior to the lateral orbital rim.

Lower Eyelid

The lower eyelid anterior lamellae structures of skin and orbicularis muscle are analogous to the upper eyelid (see **Fig. 2**).

ORBITAL SEPTUM AND PRESEPTAL FAT PADS
Upper Eyelid

The orbital septum is a critical structure of the upper eyelid, separating the orbital contents into

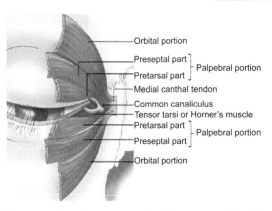

Fig. 3. Orbicularis oculi muscle. The muscle is traditionally divided into orbital and palpebral portions. The orbital portion arises from the anterior aspect of the medial canthal tendon and the periosteum above and below it. The palpebral portion is further subdivided into pretarsal and preseptal portions, each lying over the tarsal plate or orbital septum, respectively. (*From* Most SP, Mobley SR, Larrabee WF Jr. Anatomy of the eyelids. [review]. Facial Plast Surg Clin North Am 2005;13:488; with permission.)

preseptal and postseptal compartments. The orbital septum is a multilaminar fibrous sheet originating from the arcus marginalis, a fibrous line derived from the periosteum of the superior orbital rim.[6] The septum fuses with the anterior layer of the levator aponeurosis 2 to 3 mm above the tarsus. Variance in this attachment is noted and can extend from 0 to 10 mm from the superior tarsal edge. In the Asian eyelid, this fusion point can be absent or very low, resulting in the so-called single eyelid.[7] As the septum weakens with age, the postseptal fat begins to prolapse anteriorly and pseudoherniate, creating a visible bulge. These changes are important to consider when correcting the upper eyelid esthetic.

Superficial to the orbital septum, but deep to the orbicularis muscle is the adipose tissue commonly referred to as the retroorbicularis oculi fat (ROOF). This fat runs beneath the ciliary portion of the eyebrow and connects under the orbital portion of the orbicularis oculi muscle.[8,9] The ROOF contributes to eyebrow volume and mobility of the lateral eyebrow and eyelid.

Lower Eyelid

In the lower lid, the septum fuses with the capsulopalpebral fascia (analogous to the levator aponeurosis in the upper lid) about 5 mm inferior to the tarsus.[10] However, in the Asian eyelid, this fusion may be nonexistent or much closer to the tarsus.[11]

Just deep to the orbicularis in the lower lid lies the suborbicularis oculi fat pad (SOOF), analogous

to the ROOF in the upper lid. These fat pads are distinct from the orbital fat pads, which are posterior to the orbital septum. The SOOF continues inferiorly below the orbitomalar ligament, where it pads the inferior orbital rim. Ptosis of the SOOF can lead to "malar bags" and contour deformities because the inferior orbital rim becomes exposed. Ptosis of the SOOF, in conjunction with prolapse of orbital fat, can create the classic double-contour deformity.[12]

POSTERIOR LAMELLAE
Upper Eyelid

The levator palpebrae superioris, a striated muscle, arises from the lesser wing of the sphenoid in the orbital apex and extends anteriorly to become the fibrous levator aponeurosis. This aponeurosis comprises 2 separate layers: the anterior and posterior layer (**Fig. 4**). The anterior layer is thick with few muscle fibers and is reflected a few millimeters above the tarsus to become contiguous with the orbital septum. The posterior layer then travels until it attaches by elastic fibers to both the lower third of the tarsal plate and the eyelid subcutaneous tissues.[13,14] This posterior layer contributes to the formation of the upper eyelid skin crease.[15] With age, the levator muscle and aponeurosis tend to elongate, leading to involutional ptosis; this can usually be corrected with advancement of the aponeurotic attachment.

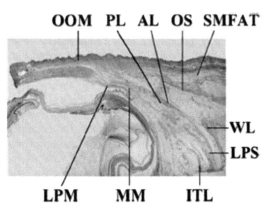

Fig. 4. Sagittal microscopic section of the upper eyelid. AL, anterior layer of the levator aponeurosis; ITL, intermuscular transverse ligament; LPM, lamina propria mucosae of conjunctiva; LPS, levator palpebrae superioris muscle; MM, Müller muscle; OOM, orbicularis oculi muscle; OS, orbital septum; PL, posterior layer of the levator aponeurosis; SMFAT, submuscular fibroadipose tissue; WL, Whitnall ligament. (*From* Kakizaki H, Malhotra R, Selva D. Upper eyelid anatomy: an update. Ann Plast Surg 2009;63(3): 337; with permission.)

The levator muscle itself is up to 40 mm long, whereas the aponeurotic distal portion is 14 to 20 mm long. The superior division of the oculomotor nerve provides innervation to this muscle and is the primary elevator of the upper eyelid. Medially, the aponeurosis creates a weak horn attaching on the medial canthal tendon and to the posterior lacrimal crest. The lateral horn of the aponeurosis is thicker and more robust.[16] The lateral aponeurosis travels to separate the lacrimal and palpebral portions of the lacrimal gland before it inserts onto the lateral canthal tendon.[4]

Deep to the levator aponeurosis lies the superior tarsal muscle or Müller muscle.[17] This muscle originates deep to the distal portion of the levator palpebrae superioris by interlacing with the striated muscles and attaches to the upper margin of the tarsus.[16] A potential space exists between these muscles termed the postaponeurotic space. This smooth muscle contributes to the resting tone of the upper eyelid, providing about 2 to 3 mm of upper eyelid elevation, and is innervated by sympathetic fibers. The sympathetic nerves travel along the ophthalmic artery and into the muscle. With age, this muscle can thin, elongate, and become infiltrated with fat.[14] Damage to the muscle or the sympathetic chain results in lid ptosis, which is a characteristic of Horner syndrome (along with miosis [pupillary constriction] and anhydrosis [absent sweating] of the ipsilateral face).

The lamina propria mucosa of the conjunctiva is located deep to Müller muscle (**Fig. 5**) and is a rich vascular connective tissue with an extensive vascular plexus just as thick as Müller muscle.[16] This layer is thought to have a suspensory effect on the upper eyelid, because it is continuous with the intermuscular transverse ligament.[18] As noted above, the intermuscular transverse ligament runs deep to the levator palpebrae superioris muscle and above the superior rectus muscle, forming a sleeve around the levator. The conjunctiva, the innermost layer of the eyelid, is composed of nonkeratinizing stratified columnar epithelium. This layer is continuous with the conjunctiva over the globe.

Last, the upper lid tarsal plate is deep to the levator aponeurosis while being attached to it on its anterior surface. Although the plate appears cartilaginous intraoperatively, it is actually formed from a specialized matrix of dense fibrous tissue. The plate measures 10 to 12 mm in height at the midline and tapers on both the medial and the lateral sections. Medially, the plate is secured to the medal canthal tendon. Laterally, the tarsal plate is anchored to the orbital rim by the lateral canthal tendon. Within the tarsal plate, meibomian

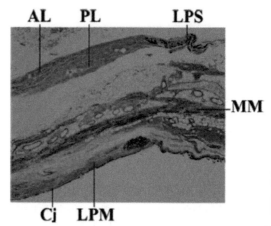

Fig. 5. The lamina propria mucosae (LPM) of conjunctiva is a component of conjunctiva and located just posterior to the Müller muscle (MM). Thickness of this lamina is as thick as that of Müller muscle and inserts onto the posterior one-half or one-fourth of the upper margin of the tarsal plate. AL, anterior layer of the levator aponeurosis; Cj, conjunctival epithelium; LPS, levator palpebrae superioris muscle; PL, posterior layer of the levator aponeurosi. (*From* Kakizaki H, Malhotra R, Selva D. Upper eyelid anatomy: an update. Ann Plast Surg 2009;63(3):338; with permission.)

glands are found. These glands secrete a thick material called meibum contributing to the corneal tear film. At the margin of the upper lid, the mucosa is tightly adherent to the underlying tarsus, and the meibomian gland ducts penetrate this area to secrete their products.[1]

Lower Eyelid

The lower lid retractors consist of the capsulopalpebral fascia and the inferior tarsal muscle, both of which ultimately attach to the tarsal plate. The capsulopalpebral fascia is analogous to the levator aponeurosis in the upper lid. It arises from the inferior rectus muscle as a dense connective tissue expansion, wrapping anteriorly around the inferior oblique muscle and contributing to Lockwood ligament, which serves as a hammock to suspend the globe between the medial and lateral check ligaments.[19] Some of these fibers also extend through the orbital fat and penetrate the preseptal orbicularis to insert subcutaneously. However, unlike the levator aponeurosis of the upper eyelid, the capsulopalpebral fascia has few attachments to the skin and so the lower lid crease is poorly formed. Although loss of the levator to the upper lid tarsus can cause ptosis, loss of attachments of the capsulopalpebral fascia to the lower lid tarsus can cause rotational instability of the lower eyelid and entropion.[20]

The inferior tarsal muscle is analogous to Mueller muscle in the upper lid. It is also composed of smooth muscle, is innervated by the sympathetic system, and lies deep to the primary retractor, the capsulopalpebral fascia. Fortunately, disrupting these muscle fibers during surgery rarely results in eyelid malposition.

The inferior tarsal height is roughly half the upper tarsus, measuring 4 to 5 mm, but is of similar length and thickness to the upper tarsus.[4] Like the upper eyelid, the posterior surface is lined with densely adherent conjunctiva.

POSTSEPTAL ORBITAL FAT
Upper Eyelid

Deep to the superior orbital septum lie the postseptal orbital fat pads (**Fig. 6**). These fat pads are traditionally divided into 2 compartments termed the central (preaponeurotic) and medial (nasal) fat pad. The central and medial fat pads are separated by the trochlea, the tendon of the superior oblique muscle, and the medial horn of the levator aponeurosis along with some thin fascial strands from Whitnall ligament.[21] Whitnall ligament originates on the superior surface of the trochlea and attaches to the lateral orbital rim under the orbital portion of the lacrimal gland.[16] This ligament, along with the intermuscular transverse ligament, which lies deep to the levator, forms a sleeve around the levator palpebrae superioris muscle and acts as a pulley for this muscle.[22]

Intraoperatively, the medial fat pad can be identified to be more pale and firm than the central fat pad. This fat pad has a significant connective tissue component and is innervated by branches of the supratrochlear nerve with a variable amount of blood vessels.[16] The central fat pad is usually deep or bright yellow, thought to be secondary to a higher content of carotenoids.[23] This fat pad extends from the trochlea to behind the lacrimal gland. A thin membranous sac encapsulates the fat containing small blood vessels and branches from the supraorbital nerve.[24] When operating on these fat pads, the trochlea separating the medial and central fat pad must be protected from damage.[4] If the trochlea is damaged, it may result in a superior oblique palsy. The lacrimal gland is located in the lateral upper eyelid postseptal compartment. This gland rests in the lacrimal fossa, which is a depression in the superior lateral orbit. Prolapse of this gland should not be mistaken for fat and accidentally excised.

Lower Eyelid

The inferior postseptal fat pads can be divided into lateral, central, and medial compartments. The lateral and central fat pads are more or less continuous, separated by the arcuate expansion, a fascial band extending from the capsulopalpebral fascia to the inferolateral orbital rim.[12,19] The central compartment is separated from the medial compartment by the inferior oblique muscle. The medial fat pad is paler and firmer in appearance and is often associated with larger-caliber vessels. The inferior oblique muscle may be encountered during removal of the medial fat pad, and care must be taken to avoid injury to this or it may result in diplopia or strabismus. It originates on the orbital floor about 5 mm posterior to the inferior orbital rim.[25] The lateral fat compartment has been observed to have more than one subsection, which can account for the persistent pseudoherniation of fat despite operative blepharoplasty.[2]

LACRIMAL SYSTEM

Tears are produced by the lacrimal gland, which is located in the upper lateral preaponeurotic compartment.[10] In the elderly, this gland can become ptotic, which may require a suspension procedure if severe. The tear film is then spread medially by a blinking action, which then enters the lacrimal system. This system comprises a single punctum at the medial aspect of each upper and lower tarsus, which is connected to a common canaliculus that drains into the lacrimal sac, which lies in the lacrimal fossa medially.[1] The lacrimal fossa is a bony groove in the nasal bone, bounded by the posterior and anterior lacrimal crests. The sac then drains in via the nasolacrimal duct and terminates intranasally through the valve of Hasner in the inferior meatus. As mentioned previously, the lacrimal sac is surrounded by the anterior and posterior limbs of the medial canthal tendon. The contraction of the muscle that occurs

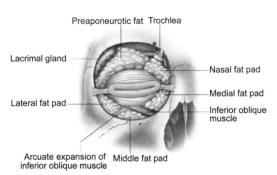

Preaponeurotic fat   Trochlea

Lacrimal gland

Nasal fat pad

Medial fat pad

Lateral fat pad

Inferior oblique muscle

Arcuate expansion of inferior oblique muscle   Middle fat pad

Fig. 6. Eyelid fat compartments. (*From* Tan KS, Oh SR, Priel A, et al. Surgical anatomy of the forehead, eyelids, and midface for the aesthetic surgeon. In: Massry GG, Murphy MR, Azizzadeh B, editors. Master techniques in blepharoplasty and periorbital rejuvenation. New York: Springer-USA; 2011. p. 16; with permission.)

with blinking creates tension on the medial canthus and compression of the lacrimal sac that creates a pumping action, which facilitates drainage of fluid into the nasal cavity.[1]

NEUROVASCULAR AND LYMPHATIC ANATOMY

Arterial inflow to the eyelids is supplied through distal branches coming from both the internal and the external carotid arteries.[4] These branches include the lacrimal, supraorbital, ophthalmic, frontal, and nasal arteries, which are all derived from the internal carotid system. Branches from the external system, including the superficial temporal artery, infraorbital artery, and angular artery, also provide some vascularity. The nasal and lacrimal arteries form an important dual-arcade system in the upper lid. The inferior-most arcade is termed the marginal arcade and is 2 to 3 mm from the lid margin. The more superior arcade, called the peripheral arcade, runs along the upper tarsal border. These arcades are important when considering blood flow to pedicled tarsoconjunctival flaps.[4] The lower eyelid arcade is less well defined compared with the upper eyelid.

Upper eyelid lymphatics are divided into a superficial (pretarsal) and deep (posttarsal) plexus.[26,27] Interruptions to this lymphatic drainage system, as frequently occurs during surgical procedures, can lead to chemosis in the postoperative setting.[28] Traditional lymphatic flow patterns map drainage from the medial portion of the eyelids to submandibular lymph nodes and from the lateral eyelid to preauricular lymph nodes. However, additional studies have suggested that parts of the upper lid, lateral lower lid, and medial canthus drain to parotid lymph nodes while the central upper eyelid and medial and central lower lid drain to submandibular lymph nodes.[26,27] Specifically, these studies demonstrate that the upper eyelid has a dual drainage system.

Sensory innervation to the eyelids is largely from the ophthalmic and maxillary divisions of the trigeminal nerve, which include the lacrimal, frontal, and nasociliary sensory cutaneous nerves.[29] Motor innervation to the orbicularis oculi comes from the zygomatic branch of the facial nerve (VII), while the inferior rectus, levator muscles, and inferior oblique are innervated by the oculomotor nerve (III). Sympathetic fibers innervate the superior and inferior tarsal muscles.

SUMMARY

The anatomy of the upper and lower lid is complex but has many analogous components. A comprehensive understanding of the interrelationships of the various compartments is important in cosmetic or reconstructive approaches to the upper and lower eyelids. The anatomic understanding of this area continues to evolve along with the variety and complexity of the procedures performed. The surgeon performing periorbital esthetic and reconstructive procedures must be aware of this complicated anatomy in order to have successful outcomes.

REFERENCES

1. Branham G, Holds JB. Brow/upper lid anatomy, aging and aesthetic analysis. Facial Plast Surg Clin North Am 2015;23(2):117–27.
2. Ridgeway JM, Larrabee WF. Anatomy for blepharoplasty and brow-lift. Facial Plast Surg 2010;26(3):177–85.
3. Rankin BS, Arden RL, Crumley RL. Lower eyelid blepharoplasty. In: Papel ID, Frodel J, Holt GR, et al, editors. Facial plastic and reconstructive surgery. 3rd edition. New York: Thieme; 2009. p. 271–3.
4. Most SP, Mobley SR, Larrabee WF Jr. Anatomy of the eyelids. Facial Plast Surg Clin North Am 2005;13(4):487–92.
5. Jones LT. An anatomical approach to problems of the eyelids and lacrimal apparatus. Arch Ophthalmol 1961;66:111–24.
6. Jordan DR, Anderson RL. Surgical anatomy of the ocular adnexa–a clinical approach. San Francisco (CA): American Academy of Ophthalmology; 1996. p. 16, 17, 26.
7. Chen WP. Asian blepharoplasty: update on anatomy and techniques. Ophthal Plast Reconstr Surg 1987;3(3):135–40.
8. Lemke BN, Stasior OG. The anatomy of eyebrow ptosis. Arch Ophthalmol 1982;100(6):981–6.
9. Putterman AM, Urist MJ. Surgical anatomy of the orbital septum. Ann Ophthalmol 1974;6(3):290–4.
10. Kontis TC, Papel ID, Larrabee WF. Surgical anatomy of the eyelids. Facial Plast Surg 1994;10(1):1–5.
11. Lim WK, Rajendran K, Choo CT. Microscopic anatomy of the lower eyelid in Asians. Ophthal Plast Reconstr Surg 2004;20(3):207–11.
12. Tan KS, Oh SR, Priel A, et al. Surgical anatomy of the forehead, eyelids, and midface for the aesthetic surgeon. In: Massry GG, Murphy MR, Azizzadeh B, editors. Master techniques in blepharoplasty and periorbital rejuvenation. New York: Springer; 2011. p. 11–23.
13. Stasior GO, Lemke BN, Wallow IH, et al. Levator aponeurosis elastic fiber network. Ophthal Plast Reconstr Surg 1993;9(1):1–10.
14. Kakizaki H, Zako M, Nakano T, et al. The levator aponeurosis consists of two layers that include smooth muscle. Ophthal Plast Reconstr Surg 2005;21:379–82.

15. Haramoto U, Kubo T, Tamatani M, et al. Anatomic study of the insertions of the levator aponeurosis and Müller's muscle in Oriental eyelids. Ann Plast Surg 2001;47:528–33.

16. Kakizaki H, Malhotra R, Selva D. Upper eyelid anatomy: an update. Ann Plast Surg 2009;63(3):336–43.

17. Anderson RL, Beard CB. The levator aponeurosis. Arch Ophthalmol 1977;95:1437–41.

18. Lukas JR, Priglinger S, Denk M, et al. Two fibromuscular transverse ligaments related to the levator palpebrae superioris: Whitnall's ligament and an intermuscular transverse ligament. Anat Rec 1996; 246:415–22.

19. Kakizaki H, Malhotra R, Madge SN, et al. Lower eyelid anatomy: an update. Ann Plast Surg 2009; 63(3):344–51.

20. Baker S. Local flaps in facial reconstruction. 2nd edition. St. Louis (MO): Mosby; 2007. p. 389–91.

21. Persichetti P, Lella FD, Delfino G, et al. Adipose compartments of the upper eyelid: anatomy applied to blepharoplasty. Plast Reconstr Surg 2004;113: 373–8.

22. Ettl A, Priglinger S, Kramer J, et al. Functional anatomy of the levator palpebrae superioris muscle and its connective tissue system. Br J Ophthalmol 1996; 80:702–7.

23. Sires BS, Lemke BN, Dortzbach RK, et al. Characterization of human orbital fat and connective tissue. Ophthal Plast Reconstr Surg 1998;14:403–14.

24. Niechajev IA, Ljungqvist A. Central (third) fat pad of the upper eyelid. Aesthetic Plast Surg 1991;15: 223–8.

25. Mowlavi A, Neumeister MW, Wilhelmi BJ. Lower blepharoplasty using bony anatomical landmarks to identify and avoid injury to the inferior oblique muscle. Plast Reconstr Surg 2002;110(5):1318–22 [discussion: 1323–4].

26. Cook BE Jr, Lucarelli MJ, Lemke BN, et al. Eyelid lymphatics I: histochemical comparisons between the monkey and human. Ophthal Plast Reconstr Surg 2002;18(1):18–23.

27. Cook BE Jr, Lucarelli MJ, Lemke BN, et al. Eyelid lymphatics II: a search for drainage patterns in the monkey and correlations with human lymphatics. Ophthal Plast Reconstr Surg 2002;18(2):99–106.

28. Levine MR, Davies R, Ross J. Chemosis following blepharoplasty: an unusual complication. Ophthalmic Surg 1994;25(9):593–6.

29. Janfaza P. Surgical anatomy of the head and neck. 1st edition. Philadelphia: Lippincott Williams & Williams; 2001. p. 170–2.

Evaluation of Eyelid Function and Aesthetics

Michael G. Neimkin, MD[a,b,*], John B. Holds, MD[a,c,d]

KEYWORDS

- Aesthetics • Face • Beauty • Aging/physiology • Eyelids/surgery • Preoperative evaluation

KEY POINTS

- The eyes and periocular area are the central aesthetic unit of the face.
- Facial aging is a dynamic process that involves skin, subcutaneous soft tissues, and bony structures.
- An understanding of what is perceived as youthful and beautiful is critical for success.
- Knowledge of the functional aspects of the eyelid and periocular area can identify preoperative red flags.

INTRODUCTION

The beauty of a woman must be seen from in her eyes, because that is the doorway to her heart, the place where love resides
— *Audrey Hepburn*

Appearance has an important role in self-perception as well as perception by others. No area is more important in self-perception than the face, which research has shown to have a profound effect on overall well-being.[1,2] As the center of the face, the functional and aesthetic importance of the periocular region cannot be overstated. Not only is the periocular area the core aesthetic unit of the face, it is also responsible for protection and function of the eye and thus the visual system. Periorbital aging changes are among the earliest to present in the face, which can cause patients distress with even small changes to this area.[3,4]

Patient attention to the periorbital region has driven cosmetic blepharoplasty to become one of most commonly performed surgical procedures in the world.[5] Although complication rates with periorbital aesthetic treatments are generally low, visually threatening events can occur. Given the intricate relationship of the periorbital area with the visual system, an intimate understanding of anatomy combined with a thorough preoperative evaluation and meticulous surgical technique are essential to provide the highest patient outcomes.[6,7] The preoperative evaluation is crucial to assessing patient goals, establishing the surgical plan, setting realistic expectations, and identifying any risk factors that could lead to poor outcomes. The following is our standard approach to evaluating the functional and aesthetic issues in the periorbital area.

THE BEAUTIFUL EYE
Symmetry

Symmetry is of paramount importance in the perception of facial beauty.[8,9] Humans have a sensitive perception of symmetry, the ability to detect perfect symmetry, and to discern very small amounts of asymmetry. The correlation between

Disclosure: The authors have nothing to disclose.
[a] Ophthalmic Plastic and Cosmetic Surgery Inc, 12990 Manchester Road, Suite 102, St Louis, MO 63131, USA;
[b] Department of Ophthalmology and Visual Sciences, Washington University in St Louis, St Louis, MO 63110, USA; [c] Department of Ophthalmology, Saint Louis University, St Louis, MO 63104, USA;
[d] Department of Otolaryngology, Saint Louis University, St Louis, MO 63104, USA
* Corresponding author.
E-mail address: mgneimkin@gmail.com

Facial Plast Surg Clin N Am 24 (2016) 97–106
http://dx.doi.org/10.1016/j.fsc.2015.12.002

symmetry and attractiveness is significant,[10–12] with studies finding digitalized mirror-image faces perceived as more attractive than the unaltered original images.[13] Thus, the importance of symmetry to oculofacial plastic surgeons cannot be overstated.

The periocular region frequently has visible asymmetry in the brow, eyelid height, amount of skin redundancy, cheek projection, and globe prominence. Although there is no general consensus on the amount of asymmetry that is clinically significant, previous studies have found significant asymmetry in up to 30% of patients.[8,14] Many patients are unaware of their asymmetries, which leads to poor surgical outcomes if not addressed properly addressed at surgery.[15] Surgeons must review with their patients, document all asymmetry, and factor its role into the treatment plan. Patients must be counseled that at least a small degree of asymmetry will persist postoperatively. Unrealistic expectations can lead to marked patient dissatisfaction.[16]

Aging

Ideally, balanced and diffuse fat distribution, a well-rounded three-dimensional structure, and good projection are hallmarks of a healthy and youthful facial appearance.[17] Little[18] described the youthful face as an ogee-shaped profile, with anterior oblique surfaces that undulate in graceful curves.

Facial aging is a dynamic process that involves skin, subcutaneous soft tissues, and bony structures. The bony remodeling of the orbit results in orbital elongation, loss of projection, and change of the bone–soft tissue relationship (**Fig. 1**), which likely contributes to the fat prolapse, hollow sulci, ptosis, brow descent, and lateral upper eyelid hooding that is commonly seen in aging.[4,19] The skin and subcutaneous tissues around the periocular area become increasingly hollow, allowing the underlying bone, muscle, remaining fat, and blood vessels to become more apparent.[17] The gradual descent and atrophy of subcutaneous tissue alters the smooth ogee curve of the youthful face.[18]

Older surgical techniques for periocular rejuvenation are generally purely subtractive, with the removal of fat and skin, which led to an increasing hollow appearance. However, the increased understanding of the aging process has resulted in the amelioration and development of new techniques leading to more successful rejuvenation outcomes.[20–22]

SKIN

Skin is the largest organ in the human body. Healthy skin tone, a smooth appearance, and brighter complexion are associated with increased attractiveness, youth, and health.[23] Because wrinkles are a sign of aging, youthful skin should be smooth. Ideally, the pigment is uniform and skin is free of blemishes with a consistent appearance (**Fig. 2**).[24,25]

UPPER EYELID

The upper eyelid margin naturally has a gently curved contour. Medially, the curve has a sharper

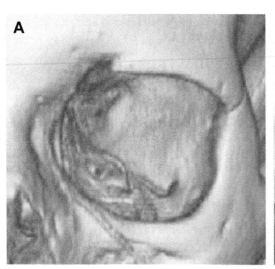
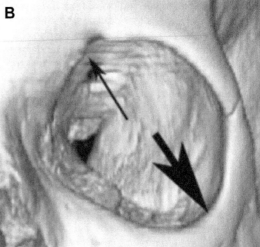

Fig. 1. Computed tomography scan of a male patient in the young age group (*A*) and a male patient in the old age group (*B*). The image from the old age groups shows significant bony remodeling (*arrows*) both superomedially and inferolaterally. (*From* Kahn DM, Shaw RB Jr. Aging of the bony orbit: a three-dimensional computed tomographic study. Aesthet Surg J 2008;28:258–64; with permission.)

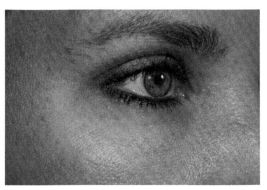

Fig. 2. Oblique view of the right brow and eyelids of a woman in her mid-30s. The skin is without rhytids or dyschromia, with uniform texture, quality, and contour. (*From* Buchanan AG, Holds JB. The beautiful eye: perception of beauty in the periocular area. In: Massry GG, editor. Master techniques in blepharoplasty and periorbital rejuvenation. Springer Science + Business Media, LLC; 2001; with permission.)

angle with the peak height located between the pupil and lateral limbus in the Western eyelid (**Fig 3**). The central height of the upper eyelid should be just below the limbus, without excessive droop or scleral show.[26] The ideal upper eyelid should not have excess fat, or skeletonization with hollowing of the sulcus (**Fig. 4**). The youthful aesthetics of the Asian upper eyelid are different in numerous

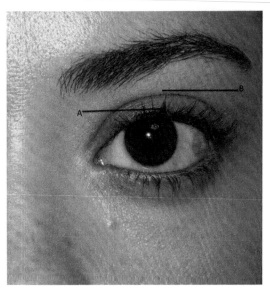

Fig. 4. (A) The superior eyelid margin is just below the limbus, and (B) the upper sulcus has no excessive fat or skeletonization. (*From* Buchanan AG, Holds JB. The beautiful eye: perception of beauty in the periocular area. In: Massry GG, editor. Master techniques in blepharoplasty and periorbital rejuvenation. Springer Science + Business Media, LLC; 2001; with permission.)

ways, including the eyelid fold, lower marginal position, and more temporal peak in the lid height.

Upper Eyelid Height

Described by Putterman and Urist[28] in 1975, the margin reflex distance (MRD) is a widely used and specific way to evaluate upper eyelid position. MRD can replace palpebral fissure because palpebral fissure does not examine the upper and lower eyelid heights independently. To determine the MRD, the surgeon shines a light held at the surgeon's eye level toward the patient's eyes in primary gaze, looking at the corneal light reflex. The MRD1 is the measurement from the corneal light reflex to the central upper eyelid margin. The MRD2 is similarly the measurement from the corneal reflex to the central lower eyelid margin. To ensure accurate measurement, surgeons must ensure that the patient's brow is in a natural position and that the surgeon's and patient's eyes are at the same level.[27,28]

Although there is variability between ethnic groups, the normal Western MRD1 is 3.5 mm to 4.5 mm.[29–31] Any asymmetry between the 2 eyes, or an abnormal MRD1, must be addressed. Many patients are unaware preoperatively and a blepharoplasty in the setting of blepharoptosis

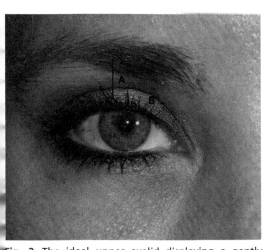

Fig. 3. The ideal upper eyelid displaying a gently curved contour. Notice (A) the peak height located between the pupil and lateral limbus just below the superior limbus, and (B) a sharper angle medially. (*From* Buchanan AG, Holds JB. The beautiful eye: perception of beauty in the periocular area. In: Massry GG, editor. Master techniques in blepharoplasty and periorbital rejuvenation. Springer Science + Business Media, LLC; 2001; with permission.)

makes the ptotic eyelid position more apparent.[32]

Levator Function

Levator function is the measurement of upper eyelid excursion from downgaze to upgaze. Ensuring that eyebrow excursion does not contribute to the levator function is key to an accurate measurement and is accomplished by manually holding the eyebrow in its normal position.[33] Normal levator function is greater than 12 mm, with an average of 15 mm. A significant decrease in levator function can indicate congenital or myopathic ptosis.[34]

Upper Eyelid Crease, Tarsal Platform Show, and Brow Fat Span

A normal, properly defined eyelid crease for white people is 10 to 12 mm above the central eyelid margin in women, and 7 to 8 mm in men. There are notable variations among different ethnic groups.[35]

Tarsal platform show (TPS) is the amount of fixed pretarsal skin that is visible inferior to the skin overlying the eyelid crease, which is normally 3 to 6 mm in Western Europeans. Brow fat span is the distance between the skin fold overlying the eyelid crease (top edge of the TPS) to the inferior brow hairs (**Fig. 5**). Attention must be paid to the symmetry of these measurements (**Fig. 6**), because TPS symmetry may be more important than MRD1 in eyelid symmetry perception.[36]

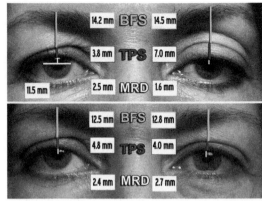

Fig. 6. (*Top*) Measurement of BFS, TPS, and MRD1 on standardized photographs (corneal diameter set at 11.5 mm for scale). (*Bottom*) In the same patient, following left ptosis surgery and bilateral asymmetric blepharoplasty, TPS symmetry has improved and BFS has shortened. (*From* Branham G, Holds JB. Brow/upper lid anatomy, aging and aesthetic analysis. Facial Plast Surg Clin North Am 2015;23(2):117–27; with permission.)

LOWER EYELID

The lower eyelid spans from the lateral to medial canthus. The lateral canthal angle is slightly higher than the medial canthus (**Fig. 7**). The lower eyelid continues with a gentle curve with the ideal position of the central margin at or slightly above the inferior limbus.[37] The thin eyelid skin transitions seamlessly to the thicker cheek inferiorly.

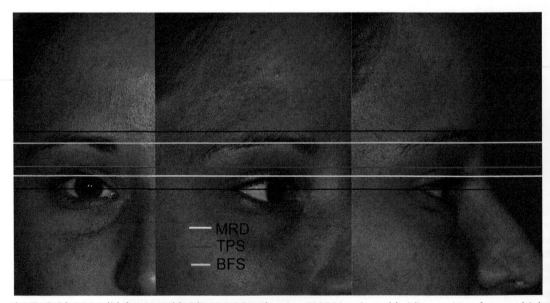

Fig. 5. Guide to eyelid, brow, and hairline position showing TPS/BFS ratio and hairline position from multiple angles. BFS, brow fat span. (*From* Branham G, Holds JB. Brow/upper lid anatomy, aging and aesthetic analysis. Facial Plast Surg Clin North Am 2015;23(2):117–27; with permission.)

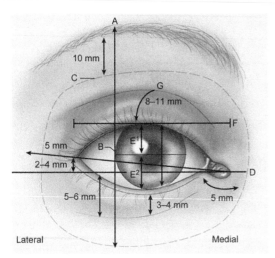

Fig. 7. Topography of the eyelid. (A) The highest point of the brow is at, or lateral to, the lateral limbus. (B) The inferior edge of the brow is shown 10 mm superior to the supraorbital rim. (C) Also shown are ranges for average palpebral height (10–12 mm) and width (28–30 mm), and (D) upper lid fold (8–11 mm, with gender and racial differences). Note that the lateral canthus is 2 to 4 mm higher than the medial canthus. (E) Intrapalpebral distance measures 10 to 12 mm. (F) Palpebral width. (G) Upper lid fold is 8 to 11 mm. E1, mean reflex distance 1; E2, mean reflex distance 2. (*From* Branham G, Holds JB. Brow/upper lid anatomy, aging and aesthetic analysis. Facial Plast Surg Clin North Am 2015;23(2):117–27; with permission.)

A small area of pretarsal orbicularis muscle just inferior to the lashes gives a healthy, youthful appearance.[38]

The transition between the eyelid and cheek, commonly referred to as the nasojugal fold or tear trough, should be a smooth, gradual transition without a hollow deformity (**Fig. 8**). Although complicated and multifactorial, a combination of facial volume loss, herniation of orbital fat, infero-lateral rim remodeling, skin laxity, and ptosis of midface tissues contributes to the common tear trough deformity seen in the aging lower eyelid.[19,21,39,40]

Laxity and Lid Position

A small degree of inferior or superior scleral show is normal in some individuals; however, any eyelid retraction must be recognized preoperatively.[37] Retraction can be differentiated from entropion or ectropion by the orientation of the tarsal plate, which should be vertical.[41] The lower eyelid should have good tone, and quickly return to proper apposition against the globe after manual distraction (snap-back test). Ectropion, entropion, epiphora, and ocular irritation are frequently associated with excessive lower eyelid laxity.[42]

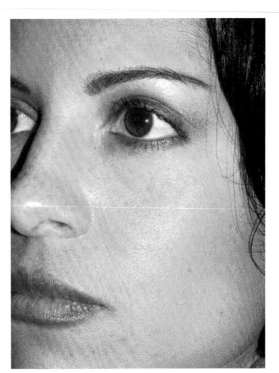

Fig. 8. Oblique view of a woman in her mid-30s. Note the smooth transition from the lower lid to the midface without contour irregularities. (*From* Buchanan AG, Holds JB. The beautiful eye: perception of beauty in the periocular area. In: Massry GG, editor. Master techniques in blepharoplasty and periorbital rejuvenation. Springer Science + Business Media, LLC; 2001; with permission.)

THE FOREHEAD AND EYEBROW

The eyebrow helps to frame the eye, and is an integral part of its beauty and perception. The head of the eyebrow is ideally positioned in a vertical line with the medial canthus and nasal ala and horizontally aligns with the tail of the brow. The female brow has a higher arc, with the maximal arch at an imaginary line drawn between the nasal ala and the lateral limbus (**Figs. 9 and 10**). The tail of the brow ideally terminates in an imaginary line drawn between the nasal ala and lateral canthus.[38]

The male eyebrow is flatter, thicker, and lower in relation to the superior orbital rim. Ideally, the male brow sits long the level of the superior orbital rim, whereas the female brow is several millimeters above the rim.[43] Eyebrow ptosis, particularly laterally, contributes to the appearance of excess lateral eyelid skin and is difficult to treat with blepharoplasty alone.[44]

The forehead is closely related to the eyebrow and eye. Its ideal width is twice the height, with a normal hairline superiorly.[45] Men may desire some furrowing of the brows, but women generally

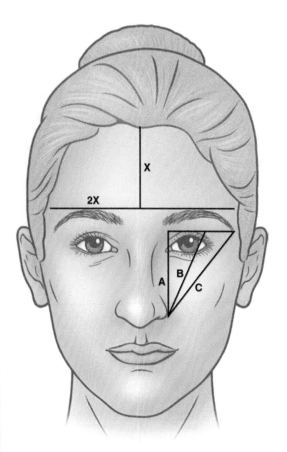

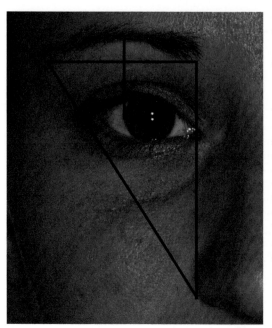

Fig. 10. Another example of the ideal brow position, showing high point of arch at lateral limbus and position of head and tail of brow. (*From* Branham G, Holds JB. Brow/upper lid anatomy, aging and aesthetic analysis. Facial Plast Surg Clin North Am 2015;23(2):117–27; with permission.)

Fig. 9. The ideal female eyebrow. (A) Medially it is in line with the medial canthus and nasal ala. (B) The peak is along a line drawn from the nasal ala through the lateral limbus. (C) Laterally it ends along a line drawn from the nasal ala through the lateral canthus. The forehead is twice as wide as its vertical height. (*From* Buchanan AG, Holds JB. The beautiful eye: perception of beauty in the periocular area. In: Massry GG, editor. Master techniques in blepharoplasty and periorbital rejuvenation. Springer Science + Business Media, LLC; 2001; with permission.)

desire a smooth forehead without wrinkles or rhytids.

CLINICAL HISTORY, REVIEW OF SYMPTOMS, AND SPECIFIC CONCERNS

All consultations begin with a detailed history of present illness, review of medical and surgical history, review of systems, and a review of medications and allergies. In addition to the standard medical evaluation ensuring that the patient is a surgical candidate, there are several specific considerations for the periocular region to minimize postoperative complications. The medical history should be meticulously reviewed for signs of thyroid disease, diagnosis of myasthenia

gravis or other neuromuscular diseases, prior surgeries, hypertension, bleeding diseases, glaucoma, and risk factors for poor postoperative healing. Aberrant regeneration following a previous facial nerve palsy is an under-recognized cause of ptosis that is often overlooked by referring physicians.[46]

Risk of Bleeding

It is important to review medications and history of any hematologic disorder to identify an increased risk of bleeding. Many patients do not understand the potency and systemic effects of over-the-counter herbs, supplements, and nonsteroidal antiinflammatory drugs. Common herbal supplements that may increase bleeding include echinacea, ephedra, garlic, ginkgo, ginseng, kava, St John's wort, and valerian.[47] Retrobulbar hemorrhage, especially with vision loss, is an exceedingly rare complication of blepharoplasty, reported in 1 in 22,000 cases.[48] Failure to control blood pressure and hold blood thinners increases this risk.[49,50]

Cataracts

In middle-aged to elderly individuals, the authors recommend inquiry of the patient's cataract status preoperatively, because cataract extraction occasionally causes postoperative ptosis. Eyelid surgery might be delayed if cataract surgery is planned in the near future.[51]

Contact Lens Usage

Inquiry of contact lens history is important, especially in the setting of ptosis. Both soft and hard contact lenses can cause ptosis via multiple mechanisms.[52] Some cases of ptosis are successfully treated medically, so ptosis in the setting of contact lens wear warrants an ophthalmologic examination preoperatively.[53,54] Patients are also warned that discontinuation of contact lens wear is necessary for 1 to 2 weeks postoperatively. In addition, a new contact lens prescription and fitting is occasionally required after upper eyelid surgery.[55]

Glaucoma, Topical Ocular Medications, and Prostaglandin-Associated Periorbitopathy

Glaucoma is a common ocular condition that is increasing in prevalence.[56] Patients with glaucoma present several potential risks to cosmetic eyelid surgeons. In patients with advanced disease potentially necessitating surgical intervention, ptosis is a common complication of trabeculectomy surgery, occurring in up to 19% of patients.[57,58] Thus, communicating with a glaucoma specialist to inquire about the patient's disease is advised.

In addition, several topical medications can affect eyelid position and appearance.

Brimonidine (Alphagan, Allergan)

Brimonidine and apraclonidine (Iopidine) are topical medications that can raise the upper eyelid. They are both alpha-adrenergic agonists that stimulate the Müller muscle, raising the lid temporarily. With a 1-mm to 3-mm elevation during use, this has garnered acceptance in aesthetic circles as a temporary medical treatment of Botox-induced ptosis.[59,60] Although apraclonidine is not a commonly used chronic glaucoma medication, brimonidine is. Clarification of a patient's continuing use of these medications and surgical expectations prevents postoperative concerns.

Prostaglandin-Associated Periorbitopathy

The low cost, effectiveness, and ease of use have helped prostaglandin analogues to become an increasingly popular first-line therapy for the treatment of glaucoma.[61–63] An early noticed effect was increased eyelash growth, which was applied for cosmetic purposes and has made bimatoprost (Latisse, Allergan) a popular option for eyelash enhancement.[64–66]

A more recently discovered negative effect of this class of therapeutic agents is a constellation of findings referred to as prostaglandin-associated periorbitopathy. Common findings include fat atrophy, deepening of the superior sulcus, decreased dermatochalasis, ptosis, enophthalmos, lower eyelid retractions, periocular edema, and thinning of the eyelid margins.[67–69] Patients using bimatoprost for cosmetic reasons have been increasingly observed to display these findings.[70] The fat atrophy is significant and may be reversible on the cessation of treatment, but can take months to years for maximum recovery.[71,72] In patients with these findings, communicating with a glaucoma specialist about switching to a different class of medication is advisable before considering aesthetic surgery.

Assessment of Tear Film and Dry Eye Syndrome

Dry eye syndrome, or keratoconjunctivitis sicca, is a common complication of blepharoplasty. Although most cases are mild and self-limited, severe cases can lead to corneal damage with associated visual limitation.[73] Failure to recognize preoperative tear deficiency can significantly worsen symptoms postoperatively.[74] Blepharoplasty is a safe operation in most of these patients; however, preoperative recognition and conservative surgical technique are paramount to ensure excellent results and avoid further exacerbations of symptoms.[75] Laser in situ keratomileusis (LASIK) surgery lessens corneal sensation, increasing the risk of dry eye syndrome and exposure complications. This history is important to elicit, and it is generally advisable to allow at least 6 to 12 months between LASIK surgery and upper eyelid surgery.[76]

Clinically, the authors' assessment includes patient history; Schirmer test with topical anesthetic (basic Schirmer); assessment of lid closure, Bell phenomenon, and lagophthalmos; and a slit lamp examination to assess the cornea.

Schirmer Testing

Schirmer testing after the application of a topical anesthetic measures the basal secretory rate, and is a commonly used preoperative screening tool.[77] After the instillation of topical anesthetic, the inferior fornicies are wicked dry and the testing strips are inserted adjacent to the puncta. Measurements of 10 mm to 30 mm are normal; measurements less than 10 mm are abnormal, suggesting the presence of dry eyes, and less than 5 mm suggests severe dry eyes.[78,79] Although the diagnostic reliability of the Schirmer test has been criticized, it remains the most commonly used test of tear production.[80]

Bell Phenomenon

Bell phenomenon is the upward rotation of the eye on lid closure, which serves as a protection mechanism for the cornea.[81] To assess, the examiner attempts to open the patient's eyelids during lid closure. If the reflex is intact, the inferior sclera visible with the globe is rotated up and out. Patients with a normal Bell phenomenon show higher tolerance to mild postoperative lagophthalmos. An absent Bell phenomenon should encourage a conservative course.[82]

REFERENCES

1. Reilly MJ, Tomsic JA, Fernandez SJ, et al. Effect of facial rejuvenation surgery on perceived attractiveness, femininity, and personality. JAMA Facial Plast Surg 2015;17(3):202–7.
2. Springer IN, Wiltfang J, Kowalski JT, et al. Mirror, mirror on the wall…: self-perception of facial beauty versus judgement by others. J Craniomaxillofac Surg 2012;40(8):773–6.
3. Bravo BSF, Rocha CRMD, Bastos JTD, et al. Comprehensive treatment of periorbital region with hyaluronic acid. J Clin Aesthet Dermatol 2015;8(6):30–5.
4. Kahn DM, Shaw RB Jr. Aging of the bony orbit: a three-dimensional computed tomographic study. Aesthet Surg J 2008;28(3):258–64.
5. Patrocinio TG, Loredo BA, Arevalo CE, et al. Complications in blepharoplasty: how to avoid and manage them. Braz J Otorhinolaryngol 2011;77(3):322–7.
6. Hartstein ME, Kikkawa D. How to avoid blepharoplasty complications. Oral Maxillofac Surg Clin North Am 2009;21(1):31–41, v–vi.
7. Oestreicher J, Mehta S. Complications of blepharoplasty: prevention and management. Plast Surg Int 2012;2012:252368.
8. Macdonald KI, Mendez AI, Hart RD, et al. Eyelid and brow asymmetry in patients evaluated for upper lid blepharoplasty. J Otolaryngol Head Neck Surg 2014;43(1):36.
9. Mealey L, Bridgstock R, Townsend GC. Symmetry and perceived facial attractiveness: a monozygotic co-twin comparison. J Pers Soc Psychol 1999;76(1):151–8.
10. Scognamillo R, Rhodes G, Morrone C, et al. A feature-based model of symmetry detection. Proc Biol Sci 2003;270(1525):1727–33.
11. Wagemans J. Characteristics and models of human symmetry detection. Trends Cogn Sci 1997;1(9):346–52.
12. Baudouin JY, Tiberghien G. Symmetry, averageness, and feature size in the facial attractiveness of women. Acta Psychol (Amst) 2004;117(3):313–32.
13. Rhodes G, Proffitt F, Grady J, et al. Facial symmetry and the perception of beauty. Psychon Bull Rev 1998;5(4):659–69.
14. Ing E, Safarpour A, Ing T, et al. Ocular adnexal asymmetry in models: a magazine photograph analysis. Can J Ophthalmol 2006;41(2):175–82.
15. Tower RN, Soparkar CNS, Patrinely JR. Perspectives on periocular asymmetry. Semin Plast Surg 2007;21(1):18–23.
16. Ellenbogen R, Swara N. Correction of asymmetrical upper eyelids by measured levator adhesion technique. Plast Reconstr Surg 1982;69(3):433–44.
17. Coleman SR, Grover R. The anatomy of the aging face: volume loss and changes in 3-dimensional topography. Aesthet Surg J 2006;26(1s):S4–9.
18. Little JW. Volumetric perceptions in midfacial aging with altered priorities for rejuvenation. Plast Reconstr Surg 2000;105(1):252–66 [discussion: 286–59].
19. Kahn DM, Shaw RB. Overview of current thoughts on facial volume and aging. Facial Plast Surg 2010;26(5):350–5.
20. Glasgold M, Lam SM, Glasgold R. Volumetric rejuvenation of the periorbital region. Facial Plast Surg 2010;26(3):252–9.
21. Castanares S. Blepharoplasty for herniated intraorbital fat; anatomical basis for a new approach. Plast Reconstr Surg (1946) 1951;8(1):46–58.
22. Bourquet J. Les hernies graisseuses de l'orbite. Notre traitement chirurgical. Bull Acad Natl Med 1924;92:1270.
23. Igarashi T, Nishino K, Nayar SK. The appearance of human skin: a survey. Foundations and Trends in Computer Graphics and Vision 2007;3(1):1–95. Available at: http://dx.doi.org/10.1561/0600000013.
24. Lee J, Jung E, Lee H, et al. Evaluation of the effects of a preparation containing asiaticoside on periocular wrinkles of human volunteers. Int J Cosmet Sci 2008;30(3):167–73.
25. Russell R. Why cosmetics work. In: Adams R, Ambady N, Nakayama K, et al, editors. The Science of Social Vision. New York: Oxford University Press; 2010. p. 186–203.
26. Shorr N, Enzer YR. Considerations in aesthetic eyelid surgery. J Dermatol Surg Oncol 1992;18(12):1081–95.
27. Putterman AM. Margin reflex distance (MRD) 1, 2, and 3. Ophthal Plast Reconstr Surg 2012;28(4):308–11.
28. Putterman AM, Urist MJ. Muller muscle-conjunctiva resection. Technique for treatment of blepharoptosis. Arch Ophthalmol 1975;93(8):619–23.
29. Small RG, Sabates NR, Burrows D. The measurement and definition of ptosis. Ophthal Plast Reconstr Surg 1989;5(3):171–5.

30. Beard C. Ptosis. 3rd edition. St. Louis (MO): CV Mosby; 1981. p. 191–2.

31. Murchison AP, Sires BA, Jian-Amadi A. Margin reflex distance in different ethnic groups. Arch Facial Plast Surg 2009;11(5):303–5.

32. Massry GG. Ptosis repair for the cosmetic surgeon. Facial Plast Surg Clin North Am 2005;13(4):533–9, vi.

33. Hui J, Tse D. Pediatric ophthalmology and strabismus. In: Wright KW, Strube YN, editors. Pediatric Ophthalmology and Strabismus. 3rd edition. New York: Oxford University Press; 2012. p. 592.

34. Frueh BR, Musch DC. Evaluation of levator muscle integrity in ptosis with levator force measurement. Ophthalmology 1996;103(2):244–50.

35. Tan K, Oh S-R, Priel A, et al. Surgical anatomy of the forehead, eyelids, and midface for the aesthetic surgeon. In: Massry GG, Murphy MR, Azizzadeh B, editors. Master techniques in blepharoplasty and periorbital rejuvenation. New York: Springer; 2011. p. 11–24.

36. Goldberg RA, Lew H. Cosmetic outcome of posterior approach ptosis surgery (an American Ophthalmological Society thesis). Trans Am Ophthalmol Soc 2011;109:157–67.

37. McCurdy JA Jr. Beautiful eyes: characteristics and application to aesthetic surgery. Facial Plast Surg 2006;22(3):204–14.

38. Wolfort FG, Gee J, Pan D, et al. Nuances of aesthetic blepharoplasty. Ann Plast Surg 1997;38(3):257–62.

39. Espinoza GM, Holds JB. Evaluation and treatment of the tear trough deformity in lower blepharoplasty. Semin Plast Surg 2007;21(1):57–64.

40. Hirmand H. Anatomy and nonsurgical correction of the tear trough deformity. Plast Reconstr Surg 2010;125(2):699–708.

41. Yanoff M, Duker JS, Augsburger JJ. Ophthalmology. Edinburg: Mosby Elsevier; 2009.

42. Liu D, Stasior OG. Lower eyelid laxity and ocular symptoms. Am J Ophthalmol 1983;95(4):545–51.

43. Sclafani AP, Jung M. Desired position, shape, and dynamic range of the normal adult eyebrow. Arch Facial Plast Surg 2010;12(2):123–7.

44. Kaye BL. The forehead lift: a useful adjunct to face lift and blepharoplasty. Plast Reconstr Surg 1977;60(2):161–71.

45. Wolfort FG, Kanter WR. Aesthetic blepharoplasty. Boston (MA): Little, Brown; 1995.

46. Chen C, Malhotra R, Muecke J, et al. Aberrant facial nerve regeneration (AFR): an under-recognized cause of ptosis. Eye (Lond) 2004;18(2):159–62.

47. Ang-Lee MK, Moss J, Yuan CS. Herbal medicines and perioperative care. JAMA 2001;286(2):208–16.

48. Hass AN, Penne RB, Stefanyszyn MA, et al. Incidence of postblepharoplasty orbital hemorrhage and associated visual loss. Ophthal Plast Reconstr Surg 2004;20(6):426–32.

49. Morax S, Touitou V. Complications of blepharoplasty. Orbit 2006;25(4):303–18.

50. Mahaffey PJ, Wallace AF. Blindness following cosmetic blepharoplasty–a review. Br J Plast Surg 1986;39(2):213–21.

51. Singh SK, Sekhar GC, Gupta S. Etiology of ptosis after cataract surgery. J Cataract Refract Surg 1997;23(9):1409–13.

52. Epstein G, Putterman AM. Acquired blepharoptosis secondary to contact-lens wear. Am J Ophthalmol 1981;91(5):634–9.

53. Bleyen I, Hiemstra CA, Devogelaere T, et al. Not only hard contact lens wear but also soft contact lens wear may be associated with blepharoptosis. Can J Ophthalmol 2011;46(4):333–6.

54. Sheldon L, Biedner B, Geltman C, et al. Giant papillary conjunctivitis and ptosis in a contact lens wearer. J Pediatr Ophthalmol Strabismus 1979;16(2):136–7.

55. Shao W, Byrne P, Harrison A, et al. Persistent blurred vision after blepharoplasty and ptosis repair. Arch Facial Plast Surg 2004;6(3):155–7.

56. Quigley HA, Broman AT. The number of people with glaucoma worldwide in 2010 and 2020. Br J Ophthalmol 2006;90(3):262–7.

57. Deady JP, Price NJ, Sutton GA. Ptosis following cataract and trabeculectomy surgery. Br J Ophthalmol 1989;73(4):283–5.

58. Naruo-Tsuchisaka A, Maruyama K, Arimoto G, et al. Incidence of postoperative ptosis following trabeculectomy with mitomycin C. J Glaucoma 2015;24(6):417–20.

59. Sadick NS. Prospective open-label study of botulinum toxin type B (Myobloc) at doses of 2,400 and 3,000 U for the treatment of glabellar wrinkles. Dermatol Surg 2003;29(5):501–7 [discussion: 507].

60. Scheinfeld N. The use of apraclonidine eyedrops to treat ptosis after the administration of botulinum toxin to the upper face. Dermatol Online J 2005;11(1):9.

61. Mick AB, Gonzalez S, Dunbar MT, et al. A cost analysis of the prostaglandin analogs. Optometry 2002;73(10):614–9.

62. Law SK. First-line treatment for elevated intraocular pressure (IOP) associated with open-angle glaucoma or ocular hypertension: focus on bimatoprost. Clin Ophthalmol 2007;1(3):225–32.

63. Linden C, Alm A. Prostaglandin analogues in the treatment of glaucoma. Drugs Aging 1999;14(5):387–98.

64. Fagien S, Walt JG, Carruthers J, et al. Patient-reported outcomes of bimatoprost for eyelash growth: results from a randomized, double-masked, vehicle-controlled, parallel-group study. Aesthet Surg J 2013;33(6):789–98.

65. Cohen JL. Enhancing the growth of natural eyelashes: the mechanism of bimatoprost-induced eyelash growth. Dermatol Surg 2010;36(9):1361–71.

66. Woodward JA, Haggerty CJ, Stinnett SS, et al. Bimatoprost 0.03% gel for cosmetic eyelash growth and enhancement. J Cosmet Dermatol 2010;9(2): 96–102.

67. Custer PL, Kent TL. Observations on prostaglandin orbitopathy. Ophthal Plast Reconstr Surg 2015. [Epub ahead of print].

68. Pasquale LR. Prostaglandin-associated periorbitopathy. Advanced Ocular Care; 2011. p. 21–5.

69. Casson RJ, Selva D. Lash ptosis caused by latanoprost. Am J Ophthalmol 2005;139(5):932–3.

70. Yam JC, Yuen NS, Chan CW. Bilateral deepening of upper lid sulcus from topical bimatoprost therapy. J Ocul Pharmacol Ther 2009;25(5):471–2.

71. Jayaprakasam A, Ghazi-Nouri S. Periorbital fat atrophy - an unfamiliar side effect of prostaglandin analogues. Orbit 2010;29(6):357–9.

72. Aydin S, Işıklıgil I, Tekşen YA, et al. Recovery of orbital fat pad prolapsus and deepening of the lid sulcus from topical bimatoprost therapy: 2 case reports and review of the literature. Cutan Ocul Toxicol 2010;29(3):212–6.

73. Hamawy AH, Farkas JP, Fagien S, et al. Preventing and managing dry eyes after periorbital surgery: a retrospective review. Plast Reconstr Surg 2009; 123(1):353–9.

74. Rees TD, Jelks GW. Blepharoplasty and the dry eye syndrome: guidelines for surgery? Plast Reconstr Surg 1981;68(2):249–52.

75. Saadat D, Dresner SC. Safety of blepharoplasty in patients with preoperative dry eyes. Arch Facial Plast Surg 2004;6(2):101–4.

76. Korn BS, Kikkawa DO, Schanzlin DJ. Blepharoplasty in the post-laser in situ keratomileusis patient: preoperative considerations to avoid dry eye syndrome. Plast Reconstr Surg 2007;119(7):2232–9.

77. Rees TD, LaTrenta GS. The role of the Schirmer's test and orbital morphology in predicting dry-eye syndrome after blepharoplasty. Plast Reconstr Surg 1988;82(4):619–25.

78. Senchyna M, Wax MB. Quantitative assessment of tear production: a review of methods and utility in dry eye drug discovery. J Ocul Biol Dis Infor 2008;1(1):1–6.

79. Pflugfelder SC, Solomon A, Stern ME. The diagnosis and management of dry eye: a twenty-five-year review. Cornea 2000;19(5):644–9.

80. Espinoza GM, Israel H, Holds JB. Survey of oculoplastic surgeons regarding clinical use of tear production tests. Ophthal Plast Reconstr Surg 2009; 25(3):197–200.

81. Wilkins RH, Brody IA. Bell's palsy and Bell's phenomenon. Arch Neurol 1969;21(6):661–2.

82. Massry G. Marking strategies for upper blepharoplasty. In: Hartstein M, Holds J, Massry G, editors. Pearls and pitfalls in cosmetic oculoplastic surgery. New York: Springer; 2008. p. 51–2.

Periorbital Surgery
Forehead, Brow, and Midface

John J. Chi, MD

KEYWORDS

- Brow lift • Upper facial rejuvenation • Ptosis • Midfacial rejuvenation • Midface lift • Aging face

KEY POINTS

- The periorbital region plays an important role in human social interactions; it effectively communicates not only emotion but also frequently the human condition.
- The evaluation and treatment of the aging face in the periorbital region necessitate careful consideration of its function and anatomy.
- There are many changes to the skin, bone, and soft tissues of the face that are associated with aging: bony atrophy, lipoatrophy, and descent of facial soft tissues.
- Many surgical and nonsurgical techniques exist to treat the aging periorbital region; however, careful consideration of the patient's complaints and existing anatomy is critical to achieving a safe and esthetically pleasing outcome.

INTRODUCTION

The evaluation and treatment of the aging in the periorbital region necessitate careful consideration of its function and anatomy. The periorbital region plays an important role in human social interactions. It effectively communicates not only emotion but also frequently the human condition. As the periorbital region is one of the first parts of the face to show signs of aging, a frequent complaint is that the patient appears tired, sad, or angry.[1]

The periorbital region is composed of the upper and lower eyelids and eyebrow. This region is bounded by the glabella medially, the forehead superiorly, the temple laterally, and the midface inferiorly. Because of the complex interplay between these facial subunits, safe and effective periorbital surgery requires an understanding of the structural changes of this region with aging and a mastery of the anatomy of the orbit, midface, forehead, and brow. The eyebrow and upper eyelid are so intimately intertwined in their function and esthetics

that they are considered 2 parts of a continuum: requiring careful consideration of one when treating the other.[2] The lower eyelid and midface share a similar relationship albeit to a lesser degree.[3–5] This article details the principles and techniques for treatment of the periorbital region with respect to the upper face and midface; the discussion of the latter will be limited to the aspects that directly impact the periorbital region.

ESTHETICS AND AGING

There are many changes to the skin, bone, and soft tissues of the face that are associated with aging[6,7] (**Box 1**). Facial aging is due to bony atrophy, lipoatrophy, and descent of facial soft tissues. The esthetic ideal for the forehead and eyebrow is a subjective and controversial topic. Because of gender, ethnic, and age-related variations, there are many published statements of the esthetic ideal.[2,8,9] Westmore's[10] ideal female brow position, one of the most popular ideal female brow positions, locates the peak at the lateral limbus.

Disclosure Statement: The author has no conflicts of interest or financial disclosures to disclose.
Division of Facial Plastic & Reconstructive Surgery, Washington University Facial Plastic Surgery Center, Washington University in St. Louis–School of Medicine, 1020 North Mason Road, Medical Building 3, Suite 205, St Louis, MO 63141, USA
E-mail address: JChi@wustl.edu

Facial Plast Surg Clin N Am 24 (2016) 107–117
http://dx.doi.org/10.1016/j.fsc.2015.12.003
1064-7406/16/$ – see front matter © 2016 Elsevier Inc. All rights reserved.

> **Box 1**
> **Aging in the face**
>
> Bony remodeling/atrophy
> Volume loss
> Brow ptosis
> Upper eyelid ptosis
> Dermatochalasis
> Lacrimal gland prolapse
> Fat prolapse
> Fat atrophy
> Temporal hollowing
> Periorbital hollowing
> Rhytids
> Skin laxity/thinning

However, current trends place the brow's peak at a more lateral position closer to the lateral canthus.[9] Given the variance in opinions, an honest dialogue between the patient and surgeon is imperative in establishing a plan of treatment that is both acceptable and achievable.

In youth, there is a smooth transition from the lower eyelid to the cheek. Ideally, the midface convexity is uniform and relatively free of concavities. With aging, there is a loss of continuity due to contour irregularities and volume differences. The bony orbital rim becomes more pronounced due to inferior displacement of midfacial fat caused by ptosis and atrophy combined with the increased prominence of orbital fat and bone superiorly. In the midface, the position of the malar fat pad is the primary distinction between the youthful face and the aging face. In the youthful face, the malar fat pad should be positioned overlying the zygomatic arch and the orbital component of the orbicularis oculi muscle. Inferiorly, the malar fat pad should be at, but not extending beyond, the nasolabial fold.[11]

PREOPERATIVE ASSESSMENT

Preoperative assessment and planning are critical to achieving safe and effective results. Prior history of facial nerve injury or weakness, neurotoxin injection, facial surgery, or trauma should be elicited. The choice of the rejuvenation technique depends on the patient's presenting complaints and anatomy, including scalp hair, eyebrow hair, hairline position and shape, forehead length, forehead shape, hairstyle, quality of skin, jowls, depth of nasolabial folds, malar contour, and degree of lift needed. There are additional considerations

that should be made when assessing the forehead, brow, and upper eyelids (**Boxes 2** and **3**). The principle of Hering's law, which describes the symmetric motor innervation of bilateral levator and frontalis muscles, should also be taken into account, especially when encountering unilateral ptosis or asymmetry.[2] Depending on the patient's needs, a combination of treatment approaches to the brow, forehead, and midface may be implemented.

In addition to recognizing the esthetic and surgical issues, a detailed history of pre-existing ocular conditions, such as prior ophthalmologic surgery, chronic lid infections, ptosis, or refractive errors, is an important part of the initial assessment. A complete medical history should be elicited to discover any comorbidities that may have ocular manifestations. The physical examination of the patient may also include visual acuity, extraocular muscle assessment, visual fields, lacrimal secretion, corneal sensation, pupillary assessment, lower eyelid position, margin gap, and the presence or absence of a Bell phenomenon. Assessment of the marginal reflex distances (MRD1, MRD2) may be useful in assessing for ptosis and ectropion. MRD1 is the distance from the pupillary light reflex to the upper eyelid. MRD2 is the distance from the pupillary light reflex to the lower eyelid. The margin gap is the distance between the margin of the upper and lower eyelid with involuntary blink and maximal effort. The palpebral fissure height is the distance between the upper and lower eyelid in primary gaze.

FOREHEAD AND BROW
Anatomy

The eyebrow extends from the glabella medially to the temporal region laterally. The skin and soft

> **Box 2**
> **Considerations when assessing the upper third of the face**
>
> *Assessing the upper third of the face*
> Brow ptosis
> Brow shape
> Upper eyelid ptosis
> Dermatochalasis
> Rhytids
> Hairline (shape, position)
> Forehead length
> Asymmetry (brow, eyelid, hairline, rhytids)
> Skin quality

(**Fig. 1**).

Box 3
Considerations when assessing the middle third of the face

Assessing the middle third of the face

Lower eyelid position (entropion, ectropion)

Negative vector orbit

Volume (bony, soft tissue)

Tear trough

Midfacial rhytids

Asymmetry (midface, eyelid, rhytids)

Skin quality

tissues of the eyebrow overly the superior orbital rim. The hair of the eyebrow is unique from that of the scalp. These hair follicles have a limited potential for growth and regeneration following injury. The hair of the eyebrow imparts much of the apparent shape to the brow: flat, arched, or sloping laterally. Men typically have thicker brows than women. The female brow is generally more superiorly located with a greater arch. The male brow is generally lower on the superior orbital rim and flatter. The brow contour may be prominent with robust soft tissue and bony contour or flat with atrophy. The muscles of the eyebrow region include the orbicularis oculi, procerus, corrugator supercilii, and depressor supercilii. These muscles are all depressors of the eyebrow and are innervated by the facial nerve. The orbicularis oculi is divided into 3 components (pretarsal, preseptal, orbital) as defined by the periorbital structure that it overlies. The procerus muscle spans the nasion to the midline glabella and is responsible for inferior displacement of the medial brow and horizontal glabellar rhytids (**Fig. 1**). The corrugator supercilii muscle spans the medial superciliary ridge to the lateral third of the brow and is responsible for inferomedial displacement of the medial brow and vertical glabellar rhytids. The depressor supercilii muscle spans the frontal process of the maxilla to the superior medial canthal region and is responsible for inferior displacement of the medial brow and oblique glabellar rhytids. The frontalis muscle is responsible for brow and

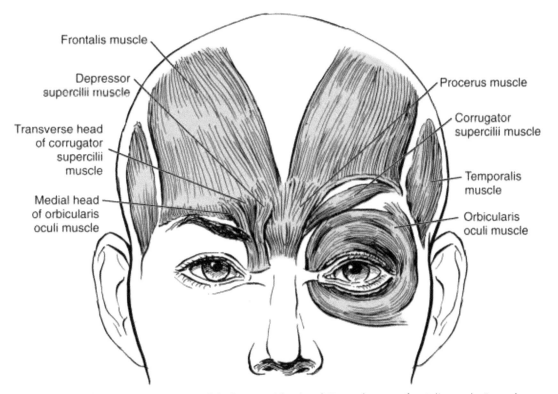

Fig. 1. Muscles relevant to rejuvenation of the brow and forehead. Brow elevators: frontalis muscle. Brow depressors: orbicularis oculi muscle, corrugator supercilii muscle (with transverse and oblique heads), depressor supercilii muscle, and procerus muscle. Other relevant muscles include the temporalis muscle. (*From* Nassif P, Griffin G. The aesthetic brow and forehead. In: Flint P, Haughey B, Lund V, et al, editors. Cummings otolaryngology. Philadelphia: Saunders; 2015. p. 432; with permission.)

forehead elevation and is innervated by the temporal branch of the facial nerve. The frontalis muscles span the galea aponeurotica anteriorly, occipitalis muscles posteriorly, and the temporal fascia laterally. Contraction of the frontalis muscle creates the horizontal rhytids of the forehead region.

The forehead extends from the superior aspect of the eyebrow inferiorly to the hairline superiorly. Laterally, the temporal region bounds the forehead. The forehead shape is impacted by the position of the eyebrows and the hairline. The average male hairline height is 6.5 to 8 cm, whereas the average female hairline height is 5 to 6 cm.[2,12] The forehead contour may be sloping posteriorly, flat, or protruding anteriorly. The forehead is composed of several layers of soft tissue: skin, connective tissue, aponeurosis, loose areolar tissue, galea, and periosteum.

Surgical Anatomy

- The frontal branch of the facial nerve provides motor innervation to the upper face. The path of this motor nerve has been well described[13–15] (**Fig. 2**). The frontal branch generally follows a path outlined by 2 points: (1) midpoint between the tragus and the lateral canthus; (2) inferior border of the ear lobule.[15]

During surgical dissection of this region, sentinel veins penetrate the soft tissues from deep to superficial at the general location of the frontal branch. At the zygomatic arch, the frontal branch remains deep to the subcutaneous musculoaponeurotic system (SMAS), but as it traverses the arch superiorly, it moves into a more superficial location. Dissection in the plane between the temporoparietal fascia and the superficial layer of the deep temporal fascia will protect and preserve the frontal branch.

- The supratrochlear and supraorbital nerves exit the superior orbital rim via a notch or complete foramen at 17.5 mm and 27.5 mm from the midline. These nerves travel with accompanying arteries and veins. Great care should be taken to preserve these neurovascular bundles during dissection. The arteries are branches of the internal carotid artery system via the ophthalmic artery. Great care should be taken to avoid intraluminal injection of local anesthetic, which has the potential for blindness.[16]
- The retro-orbicularis oculi fat extends from the preseptal portion of the eyelid to the subbrow region overlying the superior orbital rim. Removal or manipulation of this tissue should be performed with care to avoid orbital hollowing, which often exacerbates the appearance of aging.
- The conjoint tendon is composed of the condensation of the deep temporal fascia, superficial temporal fascia, and the periosteum of the periorbital region (**Fig. 3**). The conjoint tendon and arcus marginalis must be released in order to achieve an adequate brow lift.

Surgical Techniques

Endoscopic brow lift

- The endoscopic brow lift is the generally preferred surgical technique in the author's practice. The excellent scar camouflage, superb endoscopic visualization, relatively atraumatic tissue dissection, and decreased operative time make this technique the optimal choice in most patients.
- This procedure may be used with equal benefit in men and women. The forehead length is generally stable, and scalp anesthesia is minimal.
- The incisions are typically placed within the hairline: midline, 2 paramedian incisions. Two additional oblique temporal incisions are added for a lateral dissection over the

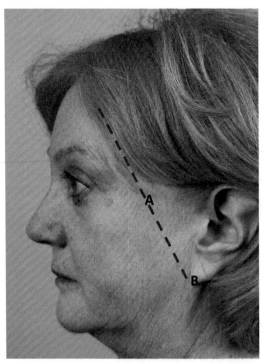

Fig. 2. The path of the frontal branch of the facial nerve follows a line drawn through 2 points: (A) midpoint between the tragus and the lateral canthus; (B) inferior border of the ear lobule.

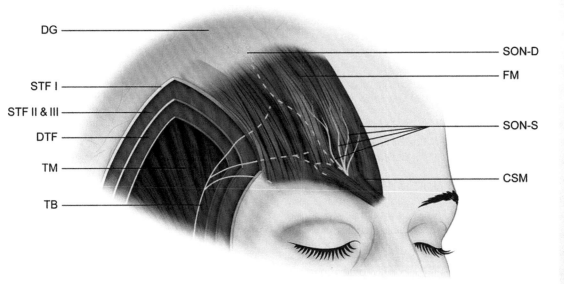

Fig. 3. Fascial layers of the temporal region. CSM, corrugators supercilii muscle; DG, deep galea plane; DTF, deep temporal fascia; FM, frontalls muscle; SON-D, deep division of the supraorbital nerve; SON-S, superficial division of the supraorbital nerve; STF, superficial temporal fascia; STF I, the superficial layer of the temporal fascia; STF II-III, the 2 deep layers of the superficial temporal fascia; TB, temporal branch of frontal nerve; TM, temporalis muscle. (*From* Lam VB, Czyz CN, Wulc AE. The brow-lid continuum: an anatomic perspective. Clin Plast Surg 2013;40:8; with permission.)

temporalis, if a temporal brow lift is to be performed in conjunction with the brow lift (see later discussion).

- The dissection is performed in either a sub-periosteal or a subgaleal plane.
- Soft tissue suspension is performed using screws (absorbable and nonabsorbable), bone tunnel with sutures, or a fixation device, such as Endotine or Ultratine (MicroAire, Charlottesville, VA, USA).
- The disadvantages include decreased precision with brow placement, the need for endoscopic equipment setup, and possible scalp anesthesia posterior to the incisions. In addition, this technique has the potential to noticeably lengthen the forehead and should be used with caution in patients with high or receding hairlines. The endoscopic visualization may be limited in patients with a round forehead contour.

Temporal brow lift

- The temporal brow lift is an excellent choice for patients with isolated lateral brow ptosis. This procedure may be performed through an open or endoscopic approach. In the endoscopic approach, the supraorbital neurovascular bundle is usually the medial extent of the dissection. The technique is otherwise

very similar to the endoscopic brow lift described above.

- In the open approach, the incision is placed at or directly anterior to the temporal hairline, and the dissection may be performed in a subcutaneous, subperiosteal, or subgaleal plane. Excess skin and soft tissue are excised from the anterior forehead skin flap.
- The disadvantages include scar visibility, alopecia at the incision, and scalp anesthesia posterior to the incision.

Direct brow lift

- The direct brow lift allows for precise control of brow shape and placement with minimal tissue dissection.
- This procedure is best suited for elderly patients with forehead rhytids and bushy eyebrows. It is also often used in patients with facial paralysis.
- The incision is placed directly at or within the superior margin of the eyebrow.
- The dissection is performed in a subcutaneous plane. Excess skin is excised from the superior aspect of the incision.
- The orbicularis oculi muscle is usually suspended to the periosteum superiorly using braided, absorbable polyglycolic acid suture.

- The disadvantages include scar visibility and possible recurrence of brow ptosis due to persistent brow depressor function.

Mid-forehead brow lift

- The mid-forehead brow lift also allows for precise placement of the brow with minimal tissue dissection.
- This procedure is best suited for patients with deep forehead rhytids or facial paralysis. It is also a good option for patients with a receding hairline.
- The incisions are made bilaterally but should not interconnect or cross the midline. They should not be linear but should adhere to the contour of a deep forehead rhytid.
- The dissection is performed in a subcutaneous plane. Excess skin is excised from around the forehead rhytid.
- The orbicularis oculi muscle is usually suspended to the periosteum superiorly using braided, absorbable polyglycolic acid suture.
- The disadvantages include scar visibility and possible recurrence of brow ptosis due to persistent brow depressor function.

Pretrichial/Trichophytic brow lift

- The pretrichial, or trichophytic, brow lift is a good option for patients who need brow and forehead lifting to address brow ptosis and forehead rhytids.
- This procedure is an excellent choice for patients with a long forehead and high frontal hairline. This approach does not lengthen the forehead, but rather shortens it and offers the potential for excellent scar camouflage. In addition, this technique offers added lift to the forehead for the treatment of forehead rhytids.
- The incision is placed at or directly anterior to the frontal hairline. The incision is irregular and beveled posterior to anterior to allow for the hair growth through the scar for improved scar camouflage.
- The dissection is performed in a subperiosteal or subgaleal plane. Excess skin and soft tissue are excised from the anterior forehead skin flap.
- The disadvantages include scar visibility, alopecia at the incision, and scalp anesthesia posterior to the incision.

Coronal brow lift

- The coronal brow lift is another option for patients who need brow and forehead lifting to address brow ptosis and forehead rhytids.

- This procedure is best suited for women with a short forehead.
- The incision is placed posterior to the hairline and follows the contour of the frontal and temporal hairline.
- The dissection is performed in the subgaleal plane. Excess skin and soft tissue are excised.
- The advantages include excellent scar camouflage at the incision.
- The disadvantages include forehead lengthening, alopecia at the incision, and scalp anesthesia posterior to the incision.

MIDFACE
Anatomy

The midface extends from the lower eyelid to the oral commissure and medially to the nose. Laterally, the superior border extends from the lateral canthus to the superior helix, and the inferior border extends from the oral commissure to the tragus. The midface defines the inferior border of the periorbital region[17,18] (**Fig. 4**). The midface is composed of several layers of soft tissue: skin,

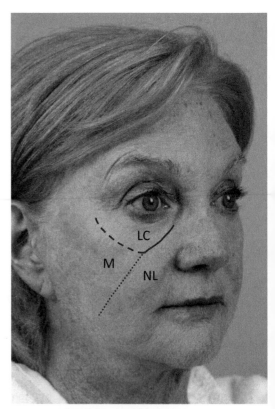

Fig. 4. The medial midface divisions (LC, lid-cheek; M, malar; NL, nasolabial) are created by the nasojugal crease (*solid line*), palpebral malar crease (*dashed line*), and midcheek furrow (*dotted line*).

subcutaneous fat, the SMAS, loose areolar tissue, and periosteum. The medial midface may be considered in the following divisions: lid-cheek, malar, and nasolabial. The malar fat pad is found in the subcutaneous layer of the midface. It is superficial and inferior to the suborbicularis oculi fat (SOOF) between the SMAS and the skin. The malar fat pad has 3 distinct components (medial, middle, and lateral temporal) separated by septae.[7] The SOOF is found between the orbito-malar and the zygomatico-cutaneous ligaments (**Fig. 5**). The SOOF extends from the medial limbus of the pupil to the temporal fat pad. The SOOF has 2 separate fat compartments (medial and lateral) and is fixed to the deep surface of the orbicularis oculi. There are 3 connective tissue bands that link the skin of this region to the bony skeleton. The lateral orbital rim has a broad band based along the frontal process of the zygoma. The orbitomalar ligament originates from the inferior orbital rim and inserts into the skin at the location of the lid-cheek junction. The zygomatico-cutaneous ligament similarly extends from the zygoma to the skin and forms the inferior boundary for the

SOOF. The SMAS is continuous with the platysma inferiorly and the temporoparietal fascia superiorly. Laterally, it constitutes a distinct tissue layer overlying the parotid gland. Medially, it transitions into a layer that joins the muscles of facial movement and separates the malar fat and buccal fat pads. The compartmentalization of fat, muscles, and connective tissues in the midface allows for the discrete functions of the eye, facial movement, and mastication.[19]

Surgical Anatomy

- The orbitomalar and zygomatico-cutaneous ligaments must be released to elevate the malar fat and superiorly displace the orbicularis oculi complex.
- Repositioning of the malar fat pad into a more superior position is critical to correcting the signs of aging of the lower eyelid and infraorbital region.
- The zygomatic and buccal branches of the facial nerve travel deep to the SMAS and innervate the zygomaticus major, zygomaticus minor, and orbicularis oculi from their deep surface. A sub-SMAS dissection should be done with care to avoid injury to these nerve branches. The levator labii superioris is innervated from its superficial surface, so any nearby subcutaneous dissection should be done with care to avoid injury to its nerve supply.
- The infraorbital neurovascular bundle emerges from the infraorbital foramen approximately 1 cm inferior to the inferior orbital rim at the midpupillary line.

Surgical Techniques

There are many different surgical approaches to the rejuvenation of the midface: soft tissue resuspension, volumization, or a combination of both. This text focuses on those approaches that address the periorbital region.

Autologous fat grafts

Midface volumization hopes to restore the youthful junction between the lower eyelid and cheek. Autologous fat grafting addresses the soft tissue volume deficiency found in the aging face with the potential for long-lasting volumization. In this technique, fat is harvested from the lower abdomen, upper hip, or any other site with abundant adipose tissues, processed, and then reinjected into the volume-deficient areas of the face. Approximately 32% of the grafted fat volume remains at 16 months.[20] Improved techniques have led to greater consistency in volumization, decreased morbidity, and increased interest

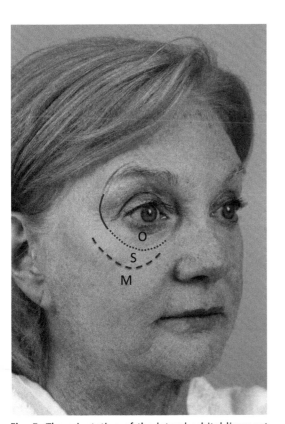

Fig. 5. The orientation of the lateral orbital ligament (*solid line*), orbitomalar ligament (*dotted line*), zygomatico-cutaneous ligament (*dashed line*). M, malar fat; O, orbital fat; S, SOOF.

among plastic surgeons.[21] Autologous fat grafting may be performed in isolation or in combination with other facial rejuvenation procedures.

Key points: autologous fat grafts

- Dimpling of the skin during fat harvest suggests that the plane of liposuction is too superficial. Harvest fat uniformly from the donor site with attention to avoid iatrogenic contour deformities. Generally, half of the harvest volume will be graftable fat: the remainder is blood, serous fluid, and tumescent fluid.
- Plan on undercorrecting the volume deficit, because it is easier to secondarily perform additional autologous fat grafting than it is to eliminate contour deformities because of overcorrection.
- In order to avoid contour deformities, instill small boluses of fat 0.03 to 0.1 mL at varying depths: supraperiosteal, midfascial to subcutaneous, subcutaneous.[22]

Alloplastic implants

Alloplastic implants are a permanent, and reversible, treatment of the augmentation of the acquired skeletal deficiency seen in midfacial aging or pre-existing congenital midfacial deficiency.[23] A distinction should be made between skeletal deficiency and soft tissue deficiency during the preoperative assessment. Alloplastic midface implants exist in several shapes and designs to improve malar, submalar, or combined deficiencies. These implants are typically made of silicone polymers, expanded polytetrafluoroethylene (Gore-Tex; W.L. Gore and Associates, Flagstaff, AZ, USA), or high-density polyethylene (Medpor; Porex Surgical Inc, College Park, GA, USA).

Key points: alloplastic implants

- Midfacial alloplastic implants are typically placed via a transoral approach with or without transcutaneous suture stabilization.
- Subperiosteal placement of alloplastic implants may result in significant and prolonged postoperative edema.[24]

Subcutaneous/sub-subcutaneous musculoaponeurotic system midface lift

The subcutaneous and sub-SMAS approaches to the midface provide efficient and effective lifting of ptotic midfacial structures. The subcutaneous midface lift allows for direct access to the ptotic malar fat pad. However, because of the superficial location of the dissection and lift, significant contour irregularities are seen with suspension.[25] A preauricular subcutaneous dissection traversing to a sub-SMAS approach ameliorates the contour deformities seen with suspension and allows for a broad vector of lifting. The incisions are usually placed in a preauricular and temporal location, so they are camouflaged well. The malar fat pad and adjacent soft tissue are then suspended via suture or fixation device to the deep temporal fascia or the periosteum of the lateral orbital rim.

Key points: subcutaneous musculoaponeurotic system midface lift

- A sub-SMAS dissection may be challenging, and difficulty with this dissection may lead to facial nerve injury.
- A sub-SMAS lift efficiently addresses midfacial soft tissue ptosis.[25]

Subperiosteal midface lift: temporal approach

The temporal approach to the subperiosteal midface lift may be performed in conjunction with an endoscopic brow lift. The incision is placed in the scalp posterior to the temporal hairline. The dissection proceeds similarly to an endoscopic brow lift and transitions to the midface via a subperiosteal incision on the zygoma. The subperiosteal dissection on the maxilla and zygoma may be performed with endoscopic or direct visualization. A sublabial incision allows for increased direct visualization, but may also increase the risk of infection.[26] The malar fat pad and adjacent soft tissue are then suspended via suture or fixation device to the deep temporal fascia or the periosteum of the lateral orbital rim.

Key points: subperiosteal midface lift

- Remaining deep to the superficial temporal fascia will ensure preservation of the temporal branch of the facial nerve.
- The infraorbital neurovascular bundle may be avoided with direct visualization or appropriate surgical dissection.
- With dissection in the appropriate tissue plane, the subperiosteal approach allows for a very safe approach to the midface.
- Significant and prolonged postoperative edema should be expected with the subperiosteal dissection.[24]

Lower eyelid approaches

Lower eyelid approaches to the midface are typically subciliary or transconjunctival. Subciliary incisions allow for conservative skin and orbicularis muscle resection with a wide exposure to the superficial and deep soft tissues of the central midface. The incision should be placed to preserve ~5 mm of pretarsal orbicularis muscle to avoid denervation and orbicularis hypotonicity.[3,24,27] Orbital fat and septal repositioning may allow for further improvement of the lid-cheek junction contour. Transconjunctival approaches are best suited for patients who do not have significant lower lid skin redundancy. However, this approach provides limited exposure, which may be improved on with a canthotomy. The plane of dissection for transpalpebral approaches may be subcutaneous, suborbicularis muscle or subperiosteal. After dissection and mobilization of the midfacial soft tissues, they are suspended with suture or fixation device to the inferior or lateral orbital rim. These approaches may be used for suspension of the SOOF or malar fat pads.

Key points: lower eyelid approaches

- The periorbital approaches allow for a vertical lift of the midface soft tissues and direct access to rearrangement of the orbital and periorbital fat pads.
- Lower eyelid malposition is a major concern with lower eyelid approaches.
- Significant dissection along the middle lamella may increase the risk for scarring of the lower eyelid.[28] Topical triamcinolone may reduce scarring of the middle lamella.[3]
- These relatively minimalistic approaches to the lid-cheek junction are best suited for patients with less severe facial aging and lower eyelid and cheek contour deformities.

NONSURGICAL TECHNIQUES: FOREHEAD, BROW, AND MIDFACE

Nonsurgical rejuvenation with neurotoxin (botulinum toxin A derivatives) or injectable fillers (hyaluronic acid, calcium hydroxylapatite, polymethyl methacrylate, poly-L-lactic acid) is the most common type of nonsurgical cosmetic procedures performed in the United States.[29]

Neurotoxins

There are 3 derivatives of botulinum toxin that are approved by the US Food and Drug Administration for facial esthetic indications: onabotulinum toxin A (Botox; Allergan, Irvine, CA, USA), abobotulinum toxin A (Dysport; Galderma Laboratories, Ft. Worth, TX, USA), and incobotulinum toxin A (Xeomin; Merz Aesthetics, San Mateo, CA, USA). These neuromodulators provide a chemical denervation of the targeted muscle by acting at the neuromuscular junction to prevent the presynaptic release of acetylcholine (**Table 1**). The position and shape of the eyebrow may be altered with selective targeting of brow depressors (orbicularis oculi,

Table 1
Neurotoxin equivalent dosage comparison

Onabotulinum Toxin A (Botox)	Incobotulinum Toxin A (Xeomin)	Abobotulinum Toxin A (Dysport)
1	1	2.5–3

From Erickson BP, Lee WW, Cohen K, et al. The role of neurotoxins in the periorbital and midfacial areas. Facial Plast Surg Clin North Am 2015;23(2):245.

procerus, corrugator supercilii, depressor supercilii) and brow elevator (frontalis). These muscles provide counteracting forces that give the brow its position and shape. For example, injection into the upper crow's feet can elevate the lateral brow due to paralysis of the lateral orbicularis oculi. Injection of the glabellar region can similarly elevate the medial brow due to paralysis of the procerus, corrugators, and depressor supercilii muscles. Finally, the brow position may be depressed with injection of the frontalis.

Key Points: Neurotoxins

- True eyelid ptosis following botulinum toxin A injection is due to toxin migration and paralysis of the eyelid muscles.
- Pseudoptosis following botulinum toxin A injection usually results from treatment of the frontalis muscle. Typically, upper eyelid fullness is present in addition to ptosis.[30]

Nonautologous Injectable Fillers

Nonautologous injectable fillers may be used for periorbital volumization.[31] Although these results may not be as long-lasting as autologous fat grafts, the improvements may last up to 2 years and typically provide a more predictable and reliable volumization. In addition, nonautologous injectable fillers may be more appropriately suited for younger patients with fewer signs of aging that may be reluctant to undergo a surgical procedure. Lower eyelid, tear trough, and lid-cheek junction contour abnormalities are well addressed with injectable fillers. The effect of hyaluronic acid products is reversible with injection of hyaluronidase, making it an excellent choice of injectable filler in the lower eyelid region.[32] The midface can be safely volumized with a variety of filler materials (**Table 2**).

Key Points: Injectable Fillers

- The periorbital skin and soft tissues are very thin. Injectable fillers administered in this region should be done with great care to avoid

Table 2
Injectable fillers in the midface

Injectable Filler	Plane of Injection
Hyaluronic acid	Deep subcutaneous, supraperiosteal
Calcium hydroxylapatite	Subdermal, supraperiosteal
Polymethyl methacrylate	Subdermal, supraperiosteal
Poly-L-lactic acid	Subdermal

From Tan M, Kontis TC. Midface volumization with injectable fillers. Facial Plast Surg Clin North Am 2015;23(2):235–6.

contour issues, fluid retention, and the Tyndall effect: a bluish discoloration due to light scattering from particles in solution.[32]

- Midface volumization with injectable fillers is more forgiving because the tissue plane of injection is often deeper and more tolerant of contour irregularities.

SPECIAL CONSIDERATIONS

- Multimodality treatment of the upper and middle third of the face is both commonplace and at times necessary to produce satisfactory esthetic results.
- For patients potentially requiring a brow lift and an upper eyelid blepharoplasty, the brow lift should be performed before performing the upper eyelid blepharoplasty so as to minimize the potential for postoperative lagophthalmos.
- Botulinum toxin A injection at the time of brow lifting may be a useful adjunct when myotomies of the brow depressors is not performed.
- Simultaneous brow and forehead lifting in conjunction with a midface lift avoids soft tissue redundancy of lifted tissues at the lateral canthus.[5]

SUMMARY

Periorbital rejuvenation requires a careful understanding of the interplay between the eyelids, brow, forehead, and midface. Reversing periorbital signs of aging requires a correction of volume loss, soft tissue ptosis, and skin changes. Many surgical and nonsurgical techniques exist to treat the aging periorbital region; however, careful consideration of the patient's complaints and existing anatomy is critical to achieving a safe and esthetically pleasing outcome.

REFERENCES

1. Shadfar S, Perkins SW. Surgical treatment of the brow and upper eyelid. Facial Plast Surg Clin North Am 2015;23(2):167–83.
2. Lam VB, Czyz CN, Wulc AE. The brow-eyelid continuum: an anatomic perspective. Clin Plast Surg 2013; 40(1):1–19.
3. Paul MD. Blending the lid/cheek junction. Aesthetic Surg J 2005;25(3):255–62.
4. Schwarcz RM, Kotlus B. Complications of lower blepharoplasty and midface lifting. Clin Plast Surg 2015;42(1):63–71.
5. Chaiet SR, Williams EF. Understanding midfacial rejuvenation in the 21st century. Facial Plast Surg 2013;29(1):40–5.
6. Lambros V. Observations on periorbital and midface aging. Plast Reconstr Surg 2007;120(5):1367–76.
7. Rohrich RJ, Pessa JE. The fat compartments of the face: anatomy and clinical implications for cosmetic surgery. Plast Reconstr Surg 2007; 119(7):2219–27.
8. Schreiber JE, Singh NK, Klatsky SA. Beauty lies in the "eyebrow" of the beholder: a public survey of eyebrow aesthetics. Aesthetic Surg J 2005;25: 348–52.
9. Hamamoto AA, Liu TW, Wong BJ. Identifying ideal brow vector position: empirical analysis of three brow archetypes. Facial Plast Surg 2013; 29(1):76–82.
10. Westmore M. Facial cosmetics in conjunction with surgery. In: Aesthetic Plastic Surgical Society Meeting. Vancouver, May 7, 1974.
11. Yousif N, Mendelson B. Anatomy of the midface. Clin Plast Surg 1995;22:227.
12. Beehner M. Hairline design in hair replacement surgery. Facial Plast Surg 2008;24(4):389–403.
13. Pitanguy I, Ramos AS. The frontal branch of the facial nerve: the importance of its variations in face lifting. Plast Reconstr Surg 1966;38(4):352–6.
14. Trussler AP. The frontal branch of the facial nerve across the zygomatic arch: anatomical relevance of the high-SMAS technique. Plast Reconstr Surg 2010;125(4):1221–9.
15. Sabini P, Wayne I, Quatela VC. Anatomical guides to precisely localize the frontal branch of the facial nerve. Arch Facial Plast Surg 2003;5(2):150–2.
16. Branham GH, Holds JB. Brow/upper lid anatomy, aging and aesthetic analysis. Facial Plast Surg Clin North Am 2015;23(2):117–27.
17. Mendelson BC, Muzaffar AR, Adams WP. Surgical anatomy of the midcheek and malar mounds. Plast Reconstr Surg 2002;110(3):885–96.
18. Mendelson BC, Jacobson SR. Surgical anatomy of the midcheek: facial layers, spaces, and the midcheek segments. Clin Plast Surg 2008;35(3): 395–404.

19. Levesque AY, de la Torre JI. Midface anatomy, aging and aesthetic analysis. Facial Plast Surg Clin North Am 2015;23(2):129–36.

20. Meier JD, Glasgold RA, Glasgold MJ. Autologous fat grafting: long-term evidence of its efficacy in midfacial rejuvenation. Arch Facial Plast Surg 2009;11:24–8.

21. Lam SM. A new paradigm for the aging face. Facial Plast Surg Clin North Am 2010;18(1):1–6.

22. Rabach LA, Glasgold RA, Lam SM, et al. Midface sculpting with autologous fat. Facial Plast Surg Clin North Am 2015;23(2):221–31.

23. Paul MD. Morphologic and gender considerations in midface rejuvenation. Aesthetic Surg J 2001;21:349–53.

24. Sclafani AP, Dibelius G. Transpalpebral midface lift. Facial Plast Surg Clin North Am 2015;23(2):209–19.

25. Keller G, Quatela VC, Antunes MB, et al. Midface lift: panel discussion. Facial Plast Surg Clin North Am 2014;22(1):119–37.

26. Engle RD, Pollei TR, Williams EF. Endoscopic midfacial rejuvenation. Facial Plast Surg Clin North Am 2015;23(2):201–8.

27. Moelleken BR. Midfacial rejuvenation. Facial Plast Surg 2003;19(2):209–21.

28. Mack WP. Complications in periocular rejuvenation. Facial Plast Surg Clin North Am 2010;18:435–56.

29. American Society for Aesthetic Plastic Surgery. 2014 Cosmetic surgery national data bank: 2014 statistics. Available at: http://www.surgery.org/sites/default/files/2014-Stats.pdf. Accessed September 8, 2015.

30. Briceno CA, Zhang-Nunes SX, Massry GG. Minimally invasive options for the brow and upper lid. Facial Plast Surg Clin North Am 2015;23(2):153–66.

31. Tan M, Kontis TC. Midface volumization with injectable fillers. Facial Plast Surg Clin North Am 2015;23(2):233–42.

32. DeLorenzi C. Complications of injectable fillers, part 1. Aesthetic Surg J 2013;33:561–75.

Upper Lid Blepharoplasty

Samuel Hahn, MD[a], John B. Holds, MD[b,c], Steven M. Couch, MD[d],*

KEYWORDS

- Blepharoplasty • Upper eyelid • Upper lid blepharoplasty • Dermatochalasis • Brow ptosis
- Periorbital aging • Lid crease

KEY POINTS

- The brow and upper lid are assessed as a continuous aesthetic unit.
- Upper lid aging is due to tissue descent and laxity as well as volumetric changes associated with bony orbital remodeling and the involution of orbital fat.
- Graded approach to upper lid blepharoplasty is important with restoration or augmentation of volume to avoid an unnatural, hollowed appearance.
- Careful preoperative planning as well as understanding and managing patients' expectations are keys to a successful postoperative outcome.

Upper lid blepharoplasty is one of the most common facial plastic surgeries performed, which can be done for functional or aesthetic indications. Successful upper lid blepharoplasty requires the surgeon to develop a clear understanding of the relevant periorbital anatomy, especially the relationship between the brow and the upper lid, as well as the anatomic changes that occur during the aging process. Current thoughts on eyelid aging involve not only tissue descent and laxity but also total orbital volume loss.[1,2] This volume loss involves both bone and soft tissue around the eye and results in brow descent, especially temporally, along with lateral hooding of the upper lid skin. The loss of brow and eyelid volume creates relative skin excess in the upper lid contributing to dermatochalasis.

Traditionally, blepharoplasty techniques focused on the excision of excessive eyelid skin, muscle, and fat. However, these subtractive techniques may result in eyelids that appear hollow and unnatural with a deep superior sulcus and excessive tarsal platform show. Contemporary approaches to upper lid blepharoplasty have evolved with more appropriate tissue resection and repositioning, aimed at restoration of the upper eyelids to appear balanced and youthful. The ultimate goal of upper lid blepharoplasty is the restoration and rejuvenation of youthful upper eyelid topography.

PERIORBITAL ANATOMY
Brow Anatomy

Understanding the upper eyelid anatomy and its relationship with the brow is crucial to performing a successful upper lid blepharoplasty. The upper lids are assessed as a continuous aesthetic unit with the brow given the intricate interaction between the brow and upper eyelid.[3] The brow is composed of hair-bearing skin and soft tissue that cover the superior orbital rim. Deep to the hair-bearing skin lies the corrugator supercilii muscle, which acts as a brow depressor along with the procerus muscle medially at the glabella and the orbicularis oculi muscle interdigitating through the area. The frontalis muscle, absent laterally, acts as the lone brow elevator. The subciliary brow transitions into the upper eyelid at the arcus marginalis on the superior orbital rim. Deep to the

---

[a] Facial Plastic Surgery, Department of Otolaryngology, Head and Neck Surgery, Washington University School of Medicine, 1020 N. Mason Road, Suite 205, Creve Coeur, St Louis, MO 63141 USA; [b] Department of Ophthalmology, Saint Louis University, 12990 Manchester Suite 102, St Louis, MO 63131, USA; [c] Department of Otolaryngology, Head and Neck Surgery, Saint Louis University, 12990 Manchester Suite 102, St Louis, MO 63131, USA; [d] Oculofacial Plastic and Reconstructive Surgery, Department of Ophthalmology and Visual Sciences, Washington University School of Medicine, 660 South Euclid Avenue, Campus Box 8096, St Louis, MO 63110, USA
* Corresponding author. 660 South Euclid Avenue, Campus Box 8096, St Louis, MO 63110.
E-mail address: CouchS@vision.wustl.edu

Facial Plast Surg Clin N Am 24 (2016) 119–127
http://dx.doi.org/10.1016/j.fsc.2016.01.002
1064-7406/16/$ – see front matter © 2016 Elsevier Inc. All rights reserved.

facialplastic.theclinics.com

orbital orbicularis muscle and frontalis muscle, the retro-orbicularis oculi fat (ROOF) fat pad provides fullness of the brow and upper lid region (**Fig. 1**). Traditionally, resection of the ROOF was considered an important adjunct in upper lid blepharoplasty. However, ROOF sculpting enhances an atrophic appearance to the upper lid, which accentuates hollowing seen with aging. Modern blepharoplasty approaches have generally shifted focus to retaining or even augmenting volume in this region.

Upper Lid Anatomy

The upper eyelid is often divided into anterior and posterior lamellae with the orbital septum separating the two compartments. The anterior lamella is composed of the skin and orbicularis oculi muscle. The skin of the upper eyelid is very thin and contains few sebaceous and adnexal structures. The orbicularis oculi muscle lies immediately deep to the skin with no intervening subcutaneous fat. The orbicularis muscle is further divided into the orbital, preseptal, and pretarsal segments. The orbital component is the outer most portion of the muscle and lies over the superior orbital rim and deep to the brow. The orbital orbicularis muscle fibers interlink with the corrugator supercilii acting as a brow depressor and opposing the frontalis muscle superiorly. The orbital orbicularis lies

unopposed laterally at the tail of the brow contributing to the involutional descent of the lateral brow. The preseptal portion of the orbicularis lies between the brow and tarsal region superficial to the orbital septum, and the pretarsal orbicularis directly overlies the tarsus. The preseptal and pretarsal components are often referred to as the palpebral portion of the orbicularis muscle and are important in active tear drainage and involuntary blinking.

The orbital septum is a thin adventitial layer of connective tissue that separates the anterior and posterior lamellae. The orbital septum lies deep to the preseptal orbicularis oculi muscle and originates from the arcus marginalis at the superior orbital rim, fusing onto the levator aponeurosis and tarsal plate inferiorly. It acts as a retaining layer for the orbital fat and is an important anatomic barrier and surgical landmark during blepharoplasty.

The orbital fat is located immediately posterior to the orbital septum and anterior to the levator aponeurosis. There are 2 fat compartments within the upper eyelid: the nasal or medial fat pad and central or middle fat pad (**Fig. 2**). A layer of thin fibrous sheet and the trochlea of superior oblique separate the two compartments. The nasal fat pad is whiter and denser than the central fat pad and can help distinguish the origin of the fat during blepharoplasty. The central fat is also called the

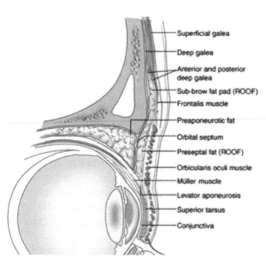

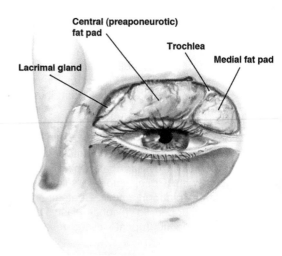

Fig. 1. Cross-sectional anatomy of the upper lids. The anterior lamella includes the skin and orbicularis muscle. The posterior lamella includes upper lid elevators consisting of the Müller muscle, the levator muscle/aponeurosis, tarsus, and conjunctiva. Note the preseptal positioning of the ROOF. (*From* Most SP, Mobley SR, Larrabee WF Jr. Anatomy of the eyelids [review]. Facial Plast Surg Clin North Am 2005;13:487–92; with permission.)

Fig. 2. Fat compartments of the eyelid. Only the medial (nasal) and central (preaponeurotic) fat compartments exist in the upper lid. The tail of the central fat pad if often tucked under the orbital rim laterally. The lacrimal gland occupies the lateral compartment. (*From* Lieberman DM, Quatela VC. Upper lid blepharoplasty: a current perspective. Clin Plast Surg 2013;40(1):157–65; with permission.)

preaponeurotic fat as it overlies the levator aponeurosis. Identifying the preaponeurotic fat in upper lid blepharoplasty helps orient the surgeon to the location of the levator aponeurosis and helps prevent unintended injury to the upper lid elevator. The lateral third of the orbit is occupied by the lacrimal gland, which normally lies within the lacrimal fossa. Lacrimal gland prolapse, however, is commonly seen with aging. The lacrimal gland must not be mistaken for fat and inadvertently excised during surgery. In the functional blepharoplasty population, moderate gland prolapse is noted in up to 60% of patients, which may be corrected with suture repositioning.[4]

The posterior lamella is composed of the levator palpebrae superioris and levator aponeurosis (superiorly), tarsus (inferiorly), Müller muscle, and conjunctiva. The levator palpebrae superioris and its associated aponeurosis is the main retractor of the upper eyelid. The levator aponeurosis inserts onto the inferior two-thirds of the tarsus with anterior fibers attaching to the orbicularis muscle and skin forming the supratarsal crease. The Müller muscle is a sympathetically innervated smooth muscle that acts as an accessory lid elevator originating from the undersurface of the levator muscle at the muscle-aponeurotic junction and inserting into the superior tarsus. The Müller muscle provides 1.5 to 2.0 mm of upper lid elevation. The tarsus is a dense band of fibrous connective tissue that acts as the structural support along the inferior portion of the eyelid. The upper lid tarsal plate measures approximately 10 to 12 mm in height at the midpupillary line and tapers across its 30-mm width. The palpebral conjunctiva is tightly adherent to the tarsus and Müller muscle and apposes the globe, wiping the cornea with each blink.

AESTHETICS AND AGING OF THE UPPER LID
Upper Lid and Brow Aesthetics

The upper lid and brow are considered a single aesthetic unit and are considered together when discussing the aesthetics and aging of this region.[3] Classic brow aesthetics suggest that the brow is situated at (in men) or slightly above (in women) the level of the supraorbital rim. The medial brow sits above the medial canthus and gently curves with the peak arch of the female brow located between the lateral limbus and the lateral canthus.[5,6] The male brow is less arched. Contemporary brow aesthetics are trending toward a slightly lower-set brow with fuller subbrow fat pad.[7] The brow should transition smoothly to the upper lid without evidence of fat protrusion or superior sulcus hollowing.[8] Traditional upper lid

metrics note an average palpebral height of 10 to 12 mm and lid crease height of 8 to 10 mm and 6 to 8 mm in Caucasian females and males, respectively. However, upper eyelid aesthetics are more nuanced and can be assessed based on the height and contour of the tarsal plate show (TPS), segment of skin exposed above the lashes in frontal view, and brow fat span (BFS), the distance from the resting eyelid fold to the inferior brow. Morley and colleagues[9] showed that a youthful appearing eye had a smooth, full upper lid with TPS:BFS ratio of 1.0:1.5 in males and 1.0:1.5 medially and 1:3 laterally in females (**Fig. 3**).

Upper Lid and Brow Aging

The aging process of the brow and upper lid is a dynamic process that involves physiologic changes to skin, soft tissue, and bony periorbital structures. The eyelid skin loses elastin and collagen resulting in skin laxity and rhytids.[10] Involution of the fat and pretarsal soft tissue causes a concomitant elevation in height in the supratarsal fold and increased skin laxity and redundancy.[11] There is temporal brow descent with aging due to volume loss and lack of frontalis elevation of the lateral brow as well as orbital fat and lacrimal gland prolapse.

There is a noted shift in upper lid fat volume with relative increase in the nasal fat pad and decrease

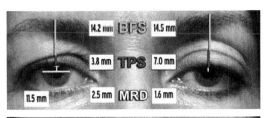
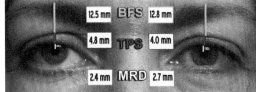

Fig. 3. Top: measurements for BFS, TPS, and margin reflex distance (MRD) on standardized photographs (corneal diameter set at 11.5 mm for scale). Bottom: following left ptosis repair and bilateral blepharoplasty, left upper lid fullness has improved, TPS symmetry has improved, and BFS has shortened; ratio of TPS:BFS approximately 1:3. (*From* Goldberg RA, Lew H. Cosmetic outcome of posterior approach ptosis surgery (an American Ophthalmologic Society thesis). Trans Am Ophthalmol Soc 2011;109:159; republished with permission of the American Ophthalmological Society.)

in the preaponeurotic fat pad with aging.[12] As the preaponeurotic fat involutes and retracts, the upper lid sulcus deepens and the supratarsal crease elevates. These changes contribute to the typical medial fat herniation and central hollowing of the aged eye or so-called A-frame deformity. Additionally, volume loss in the surrounding facial fat compartments contributes to the aged appearance of the upper lid.[2]

Bony changes involving the orbit and surrounding facial skeleton also occur with normal aging. Pessa and Chen[13] describe an increase in size of the orbital aperture along the superomedial and inferolateral dimension leading to prominence of the medial fat pad superiorly and tear trough inferiorly. The loss of bony support under the brow may contribute to further brow ptosis due to subbrow volume loss.[14]

As our understanding in both the aesthetics of a youthful-appearing eye and the aging process that alters this appearance expand, blepharoplasty techniques have shifted from a subtractive approach to one that balances appropriate excision with periorbital volume restoration and augmentation. Blepharoplasty surgeons must carefully evaluate each patient and determine the degree of tissue resection or volume preservation/augmentation that is indicated with each procedure.

PREOPERATIVE ASSESSMENT FOR UPPER LID BLEPHAROPLASTY

Determining patients' candidacy for upper lid blepharoplasty requires a thorough review of their medical and ophthalmologic history, careful examination of their brow and upper eyelid, as well as a candid discussion regarding patients' expectations from surgery.

Medical History

Preoperative assessment starts with a thorough medical and ophthalmologic history to identify potential risks for undergoing upper lid blepharoplasty. The surgeon should elicit a history of dry eyes, prior eyelid surgery, vision correction surgery (eg, laser-assisted in situ keratomileusis, photorefractive keratectomy), history of eye trauma, glaucoma, blepharitis, and thyroid diseases (eg, Graves disease). In patients presenting with dry eyes, the utility of Schirmer testing is controversial and the condition may warrant an autoimmune workup and formal rheumatologic and ophthalmologic evaluation.[15]

Other medical comorbidities, including uncontrolled hypertension, coagulopathy or bleeding disorder, active use of antiplatelet or anticoagulant agents, and autoimmune disease, may serve as relative contraindications to surgery.

Examination of Upper Lid and Brow

As discussed previously, the brow and upper eyelid are evaluated collectively during any consultation for upper lid blepharoplasty. Careful evaluation of brow position and symmetry is noted. Oftentimes, patients seeking blepharoplasty for apparent dermatochalasis demonstrate brow ptosis as the primary defect. Manual repositioning of the brow to the correct anatomic location at or above the supraorbital rim will allow for accurate assessment of the upper lid. Patients must understand that a brow lift alone or in conjunction with upper lid blepharoplasty may be necessary to achieve the desired aesthetic result.

Examination of the upper lid also assesses for upper lid position and symmetry. Preexisting asymmetry or ptosis may not be apparent to patients and can be masked by the aging process. The standard measurement used to determine the upper lid position is the margin reflex distance-1 (MRD-1), the distance from the corneal light reflex to the upper lid margin while in primary gaze. MRD-1 measurement of less than 2.5 mm or the upper lid margin vertically covering greater than 2 mm of the superior limbus is suggestive of blepharoptosis. Patients are assessed for lid excursion from an extreme down gaze to an extreme up gaze. If lid excursion is normal ($\geq$12 mm), the ptosis is most likely secondary to dehiscence of the levator aponeurosis.

Familiarity with the Hering law of equal innervation is important for surgeons performing blepharoplasty with brow or lid ptosis or significant dermatochalasis. If visual obstruction from ptosis or significant dermatochalasis is present, the muscle tone of the levator palpebrae superioris and/or frontalis muscle is increased to elevate the eyelid.[3] Patients with blepharoptosis often present with compensatory brow elevation. This compensatory hyperactivity of the frontalis muscle is evidenced by increased horizontal forehead rhytids. It is essential to examine patients with the frontalis muscle relaxed to accurately determine brow position and the presence of lid ptosis. Correction of the visual obstruction diminishes the afferent input to the frontalis and levator muscles, resulting in muscle relaxation revealing the underlying brow or lid ptosis.[8] Patients with blepharoptosis may need to be referred to an oculofacial plastic surgeon for management.

A complete preoperative evaluation also includes assessment of globe position, Bell phenomenon, facial nerve function, visual acuity, and visual field testing. A formal ophthalmologic evaluation is warranted for any concerning findings.

Preoperative Surgical Planning

Preoperative surgical planning is performed with the brow elevated to minimize the effect of brow skin and soft tissue on the upper lid. The supratarsal lid crease can be measured using a ruler or calipers. Classic measurements of the lid crease height are 8 to 10 mm for females and 6 to 8 mm for males. Redundant upper lid skin is gently pinched to approximate the planned excision and observe for lid margin rotation or elevation. It is important to delineate upper lid skin from brow skin as resection of brow skin may lead to lagophthalmos, a high unnatural supratarsal crease, and unsightly scarring.

Preoperative Photography

Standardized preoperative photographs are performed for any patient interested in blepharoplasty or other facial surgery. Photographs include frontal views of the eyes. Photographs in primary, up, and down gaze will assist not only with preoperative planning but also serve as an important communication tool with patients, especially if they have baseline asymmetry or brow or lid ptosis.

Clear communication with patients regarding their desired changes and realistic treatment expectations based on preoperative assessment is necessary for a positive outcome. As with all surgery, understanding and managing patients' expectations are paramount.

SURGICAL TECHNIQUE

Patients are marked before any distortion of skin by local anesthetics. Patients are seated in an upright position in primary gaze and with their eyes gently closed (**Fig. 4**). The brows are elevated just to the point of eyelash lifting to allow full visualization of the upper lid skin and natural supratarsal crease. The supratarsal crease is apparent as the first crease over the tarsus. In older individuals, the crease may be indistinct. The supratarsal crease is marked medially from the level of the puncta, across the eyelid, and up to the lateral orbital rim (up to 1.5 cm from the lateral canthal angle).

If the crease is indistinct or elevated as with blepharoptosis, the central eyelid crease incision line is appropriately marked between 8 and 10 mm (women) and 6 and 8 mm (men) from the lid margin. Patients with a smaller crowded orbital aperture benefit from lower eyelid creases, and those with large orbital openings have a more

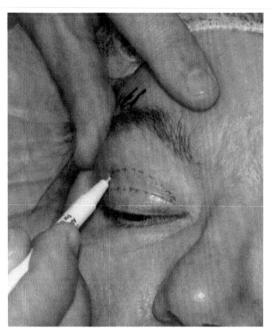

Fig. 4. Preoperative upper lid marking is performed with patient in an upright-seated position.

aesthetically pleasing result with higher creases. The crease is gently curved superiorly with an approximately 2-mm and 1-mm decrease in crease height at the medial and lateral aspects, respectively. Traditionally, a safety parameter to allow eyelid closure following blepharoplasty is to leave a minimum of 20 mm of skin between the inferior aspect of the brow and the eyelid margin. Pinch testing will also confirm appropriate amounts of skin excision to prevent lagophthalmos. If simultaneous brow lifting procedures are performed, blepharoplasty markings are reconfirmed after the brows are lifted intraoperatively.

Following blepharoplasty marking, the eyelid is infiltrated with local anesthesia containing epinephrine and a full-face preparation is performed. Sterile draping is performed to expose the entire face. Corneal protective shields are recommended before incision. Skin incision is made using a steel or diamond blade, needle-tipped radiofrequency or electrocautery device, or laser. Skin excision is performed as a single layer or, after gaining experience, along with an en bloc partial orbicularis muscle excision. Strategic orbicularis muscle resection is performed mostly from the central aspect of the blepharoplasty wound, leaving the orbicularis muscle intact in the medial and lateral wound bed along with an intact strip of the pretarsal orbicularis. In patients with dry eyes, consideration is given for leaving the orbicularis muscle undisturbed with lesser amount of skin excision (**Fig. 5**).

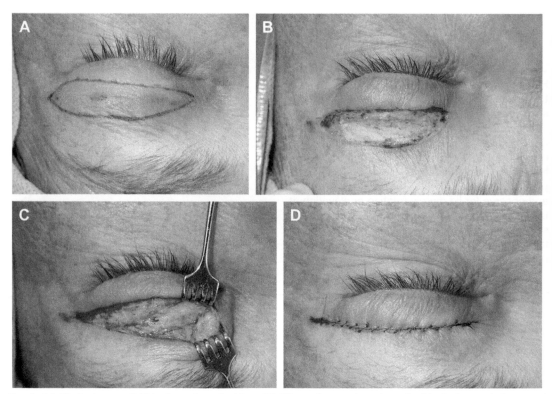

Fig. 5. (*A*) Marked upper lid blepharoplasty incision. (*B*) Skin and central portion of orbicularis muscle is excised exposing the orbital septum. (*C*) Orbital septum is incised, and orbital fat is exposed. (*D*) Blepharoplasty incision is closed with 7-0 polypropylene (Prolene) suture in a running fashion.

The orbital septum is then identified and opened as indicated to allow access to the central or medial fat. Additional local anesthetic may need to be injected into the fat pads before excision. Fat excision from the middle and nasal fat compartments are tailored to each patient. Balloting the globe can help identify the location of fat pads. Meticulous hemostasis is important, and generous cautery is applied. Newer techniques focus on preservation of the fat in the eyelid, especially the central fat pad. The medial fat pad can either be modestly excised or, in some cases of central eyelid hollowness, transposed into the central fat compartment. It is generally prudent to excise or reposition the most lateral fat from the central pad leaving the remainder of the pad undisturbed (**Fig. 6**A–E). Many patients benefit from some excision of medial fat. Care should be taken not to injure the levator aponeurosis underneath the central fat pad.

Eyelid crease fixation is important, and a precise surgical adhesion defines the exact junction in which the fixated pretarsal skin abuts the looser skin superiorly. Creation of this pretarsal platform is especially important in aesthetically oriented women for makeup placement and in older patients who typically lose their crease as they age.

A soft crease fixation is performed by capturing the levator aponeurosis with running or interrupted sutures during the eyelid closure. A more distinct crease can be created with a hard crease fixation by excising a small strip of preaponeurotic fascia and directly fixating the pretarsal orbicularis muscle to this distinct aponeurotic edge using a 7-0 vicryl suture, before wound closure. After appropriate hemostasis, the blepharoplasty wound can be closed using multiple different techniques using absorbable or nonabsorbable sutures (**Fig. 7**).

POSTOPERATIVE CARE

Wound care with topical ophthalmic antibiotic ointment is important and is used in the eyes of patients with ocular irritation. Cold compresses or ice will lessen postoperative swelling. Patients are educated on what to expect following surgery and instructed to call with significant concerns relating to pain, bleeding, unusual swelling, or visual loss.

COMPLICATIONS AND PITFALLS

Complications from upper lid blepharoplasty are usually minor, and careful surgical planning and

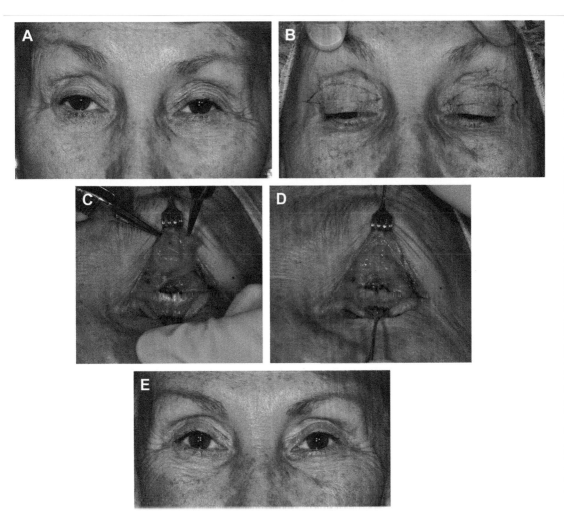

Fig. 6. (*A*) Patient with involutional aging changes of the upper lid with blepharoptosis. (*B*) Preoperative marking for upper lid blepharoplasty and ptosis repair, note the marked superior sulcus hollowing over central upper lid. (*C*) Orbital fat released from central fat compartment for transposition. Concomitant ptosis repair was performed. (*D*) Transposed fat secured to undisturbed preaponeurotic fat. (*E*) Two-month postoperative photograph demonstrating improved upper lid contour and position. Often patients with significant involution of the central fat pad can remain volume depleted despite augmentation with fat transposition.

meticulous technique can prevent most complications. Although uncommon, serious complications need to be recognized early and managed appropriately to prevent devastating outcomes.

Vision Loss

Vision loss is the most significant complication seen after upper lid blepharoplasty. There have

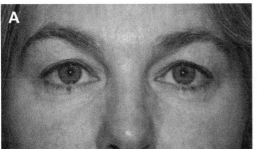
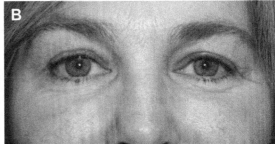

Fig. 7. Before (*A*) and after (*B*) upper lid blepharoplasty.

been reports of vision loss following upper lid blepharoplasty due to posterior optic neuropathy and inadvertent ocular injury during surgery.[16,17] However, retrobulbar hemorrhage is the most common cause of vision loss following blepharoplasty. Haas and colleagues[18] reported an incidence of retrobulbar hemorrhage of 0.05% and subsequent permanent vision loss of 0.0045%.

Retrobulbar Hemorrhage

Retrobulbar hemorrhage is most likely to occur in the first 2 to 3 hours after surgery with risk factors including hypertension, use of perioperative anticoagulation/antiplatelet medication, postoperative emesis, and increased physical activity.[18] Examination findings include proptosis, severe orbital pain, chemosis, ophthalmoplegia, and conjunctival hemorrhage. Decreased visual acuity and an afferent pupillary defect should raise concern for orbital compartment syndrome and significantly elevated intraocular pressure. Experimental models show irreversible optic nerve damage occurs within 2 hours of retinal artery occlusion.[19]

Initial management of retrobulbar hemorrhage includes releasing the sutures and opening the incision. The surgical site may be explored and any active bleeding vessels cauterized. Intravenous steroids and mannitol may be administered to lower intraocular pressure. A lateral canthotomy and cantholysis is performed to immediately reduce intraocular pressure for impending or progressive visual loss.

Eyelid Malposition: Lagophthalmos and Ptosis

Lid malposition is a challenging complication following upper lid blepharoplasty. Lagophthalmos noted early postoperatively often resolves if less than 2 to 3 mm are noted. This complication is usually due to postoperative edema and reversible denervation. Conservative treatment using ocular lubricants and taping of the eyelids at night may suffice until the lagophthalmos resolves. However, lagophthalmos or ectropion due to excessive skin excision or septal scarring may require secondary treatment for correction. Reconstruction of the anterior lamella with a full-thickness skin graft or release of septal adhesions may be necessary in severe cases. Revision blepharoplasty, concomitant brow lifting, and prominent globes should be recognized as predisposing factors for lagophthalmos or ectropion of the upper lid.

Blepharoptosis following upper lid blepharoplasty can occur because of edema or ecchymosis, which should resolve with conservative management. Inadvertent injury or interruption of the levator muscle or aponeurosis may lead to delayed or incomplete recovery of levator function. If persistent ptosis is present, ptosis repair is warranted. It is important to note any preexisting ptosis with proper photographic documentation and discuss with patients before surgery to prevent a misunderstanding postoperatively.

Dry Eyes

Ocular irritation from dry eyes and decreased blink is a common issue following upper lid blepharoplasty. Limited orbicularis resection may be prudent in patients with known dry eye syndrome. Upper lid edema and trauma from the surgery disrupts normal tear production and orbicularis function. Patients are treated with ophthalmic lubricants and artificial tears. In patients with preexisting keratoconjunctivitis sicca or related conditions, care should be taken during surgery to minimize orbicularis disruption. Persistent dry eyes following surgery may require formal ophthalmologic evaluation.

Incision-Related Issues

With proper design and closure, upper blepharoplasty incisions usually heal excellently. However, there are several potential issues that may arise related to wound healing, including wound dehiscence, hypertrophic scarring, medial webbing, and pigmentary changes. Wound dehiscence usually occurs laterally along the thicker skin when the incision is closed with a running suture. This complication may be avoided with additional interrupted sutures and closer spacing of the running suture along the incision at time of closure.

Hypertrophic scarring on the upper eyelid is rare. If the incision remains raised and firm following blepharoplasty, gentle massage of the incision may help soften the scar. Intralesional injection of steroid (triamcinolone 5 mg/mL) or 5-fluorouracil 50 mg/mL may be useful to treat for more prominent scarring or keloids.

Medial canthal webbing can occur if the incision extends medially past the medial puncta or if excessive skin is removed along the medial edge of the incision. Factors associated with excessive scarring, such as excessive cautery, predispose to wound contracture. If sizable upper lid skin resection is planned, an M-plasty or Z-plasty of the medial incision should be considered. Webbing can be corrected with transposition or V-to-Y advancement flap.[7]

Temporary hyperpigmentation of the incision line may occur because of hemosiderin deposition along the incision; or postinflammatory hyperpigmentation of the incision may occur, especially in darker-skinned patients (Fitzpatrick III and higher). Topical hydroquinone may be helpful for treatment of hyperpigmentation.

SUMMARY

Upper lid blepharoplasty is a rewarding surgical procedure for rejuvenation and restoration of the periorbital region. Understanding the relationship of the brow-lid aesthetic unit as well as current thoughts on periorbital aging and perception of aesthetics are all critical to performing effective surgery. However, understanding patients' desired aesthetic and functional changes and providing realistic expectations is paramount to delivering a successful outcome that is rewarding to patients and the surgeon.

REFERENCES

1. Bartlett SP, Grossman R, Whitaker LA. Age-related changes of the craniofacial skeleton: an anthropometric and histologic analysis. Plast Reconstr Surg 1992;90(4):592–600.
2. Rohrich RJ, Pessa JE. The fat compartments of the face: anatomy and clinical implications for cosmetic surgery. Plast Reconstr Surg 2007;120(5):1367–77.
3. Lam VB, Czyz CN, Wulc AE. The brow-lid continuum: an anatomic perspective. Clin Plast Surg 2013;40:1–19.
4. Massry GG. Prevalence of lacrimal gland prolapse in the functional blepharoplasty population. Ophthal Plast Reconstr Surg 2011;27:410–3.
5. Westmore M. Facial cosmetics in conjunction with surgery. Presented at Aesthetic Plastic Surgical Society Meeting. Vancouver (Canada), May 7, 1974.
6. Whitaker LA, Morales L Jr, Farkas LG. Aesthetic surgery of the supraorbital ridge and forehead structures. Plast Reconstr Surg 1986;78(1):23–32.
7. Rohrich RJ. Current concepts in aesthetic upper blepharoplasty. Plast Reconstr Surg 2004;113(3):32–42.
8. Branham G, Holds JB. Brow/upper lid anatomy, aging, and aesthetic analysis. Facial Plast Surg Clin North Am 2015;23(2):117–27.
9. Morley AM, Taban M, Malhotra R, et al. Use of hyaluronic acid gel for upper eyelid filling and contouring. Ophthal Plast Reconstr Surg 2009;25:440–4.
10. Pottier F, El-Shazly NZ, El-Shazly AE. Aging of orbicularis oculi: anatomophysiologic consideration in upper blepharoplasty. Arch Facial Plast Surg 2008;10(5):346–9.
11. Pepper JP, Moyer JS. Upper blepharoplasty: the aesthetic ideal. Clin Plast Surg 2013;40:133–8.
12. Korn BS, Kikkawa DO, Hicok KC. Identification and characterization of adult stem cells from human orbital adipose tissue. Ophthal Plast Reconstr Surg 2009;25:27–32.
13. Pessa JE, Chen Y. Curve analysis of the aging orbital aperture. Plast Reconstr Surg 2002;100(2):751–5.
14. Knize DM. An anatomically based study of the mechanism of eyebrow ptosis. Plast Reconstr Surg 1996;97(7):1321–33.
15. Friedland JA, Lalonde DH, Rohrich RJ. An evidence based approach to blepharoplasty. Plast Reconstr Surg 2010;126(6):2222–9.
16. Kordic H, Flammer J, Mironow A, et al. Perioperative posterior ischemic optic neuropathy as a rare complication of blepharoplasty. Ophthalmologica 2005;291(3):185–8.
17. Parikh M, Kwon YH. Vision loss after inadvertent corneal perforation during lid anesthesia. Ophthal Plast Reconstr Surg 2011;27(5):141–2.
18. Hass AN, Penne RB, Stefanyszyn MA, et al. Incidence of post-blepharoplasty orbital hemorrhage and associated visual loss. Ophthal Plast Reconstr Surg 2004;20(6):426–32.
19. Hayreh SS, Jonas JB. Optic disk and retinal nerve fiber layer damage after transient central retinal artery occlusion: an experimental study in rhesus monkeys. Am J Ophthalmol 2000;129:786–95.

Lower Eyelid Blepharoplasty

Gregory H. Branham, MD*

KEYWORDS

- Transconjunctival blepharoplasty • Lower lid laxity • Transcutaneous blepharoplasty
- Pseudoherniated fat • Tear trough deformity • Deramtochalasis • Festoon
- Orbital retaining ligament

KEY POINTS

- Incisions and flap elevation should be performed in a manner to prevent postoperative lid malposition taking care to preserve the pretarsal orbicularis muscle sling.
- Fat excision should be conservative to avoid skeletonizing the eye. Volume can be restored to the lid/cheek by fat transposition, fat autografts, and injectable filler materials.
- Orbicularis, suborbicularis oculi fat, and other lateral suspension techniques can be used to correct aging changes in the lateral lid/cheek junction.
- Conservative skin excision via subciliary approach can correct lower lid dermatochalasis.
- Aging changes associated with the medial lower lid require different approaches than the lateral lower lid.

INTRODUCTION

Lower eyelid blepharoplasty involves a complex set of maneuvers to rejuvenate the lower lid/cheek complex. The choice of which techniques to use depends on an accurate analysis of each patient's presenting problems. Ultimate success with the chosen techniques for a specific patient relies on knowledge of the relevant anatomy and meticulous execution of the surgical plan.

As we age, the brow descends and the distance from the brow/lid junction to the upper lid margin decreases, causing the eye to close in and present a tired and angry appearance. In the midface, the cheek descends and the distance from the lower lid margin to the lid/cheek junction increases resulting in a loss of the smooth transition from lid to cheek and isolation of these facial subunits.[1,2] In lower lid blepharoplasty, the surgeon is attempting to reverse aging and gravitational changes in the lid/cheek complex with a goal to shorten that distance and suspend tissues, whereas in the upper lid the goal is to lengthen the distance from the brow to the lid margin, which decreases with time. Just as in upper eye rejuvenation the brow must be addressed, so in lower eye rejuvenation the cheek/malar area must be addressed. In both, volume restoration is critical to the overall rejuvenation plan.[3] The skin texture changes that occur with age in the lower lid present an additional issue and these must be addressed as well. Smooth skin is as important as other factors in determining the perception of youthfulness and beauty.[4,5] Although this article focuses on lower eyelid rejuvenation and it is convenient to divide it in this manner, the entire periorbital area including brow and midface must be viewed and addressed as a whole.

Disclosures: The author has no disclosures or conflicts.
Facial Plastic and Reconstructive Surgery, Department of Otolarynogology-Head and Neck Surgery, Washington University School of Medicine, St Louis, MO, USA
* Facial Plastic Surgery Center, 1020 North Mason Road, Suite 205, Creve Coeur, MO 63141.
E-mail address: Branhamg@wustl.edu

facialplastic.theclinics.com

AGING CHANGES OF THE LOWER LID AND CHEEK

In youth, there is a smooth transition from the lid to the cheek with a full malar mound and a single convexity. There is no demarcation between the midface and lower lids and the skin is smooth. As we age, the changes that occur combine to create a vertically elongated lower eyelid, ptotic malar/cheek complex, a lax lower eyelid and protrusion of orbital fat. Each of these changes can be attributed to specific changes in the supporting ligaments and tissues of the face and eyes (**Fig. 1**). The orbicularis oculi muscle (OOM) is composed of a palpebral portion, which consists of pretarsal and preseptal components and an orbital component. The pretarsal component lies just anterior to the tarsus, which in the lower lid measures approximately 4 mm. The preseptal component begins at the inferior border of the tarsus and transitions to the orbital component at the arcus marginalis or orbital rim (**Fig. 2**). Medially, the tear trough or nasojugal groove is formed owing to the attachment of the orbicularis to the orbital bone just below the

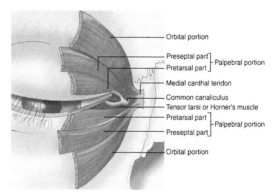

Fig. 2. Components of orbicularis oculi muscle (OOM). The OOM is composed of 3 parts. The pretarsal segment that overlies the lower tarsus measures approximately 4 mm. The preseptal segment overlies the orbital septum and extends from the inferior border of the tarsus to the arcus marginalis. The preseptal and pretarsal segments are collectively referred to as the palpebral portion of the OOM. The orbital portion of the OOM extends inferiorly from the arcus marginalis and overlies the bone. (*From* Most S, Mobley S, Larrabee W. Anatomy of the eyelids. Facial Plast Surg Clin North Am 2005;13:487–92; with permission.)

orbital rim without an intervening ligamentous structure (**Fig. 3**). Laterally, the orbicularis is attached to the bone via the orbital retaining ligament.

By measuring the lid length in individuals at every decade from their 20s to their 90s, Fezza and colleagues[6] have shown that there is a steady linear increase in lid length as measured from the lid margin to the orbital rim. The greatest change was noted in patients in their 40s. Bone loss in the periorbital and malar regions contributes to the overall volume loss associated with aging and loss of projection of the orbital rim[7] (**Fig. 4**). The orbital septum weakens, orbicularis atrophies, and the skin becomes lax with time and allows orbital fat to pseudoherniate outside the bounds of the orbital rim.[8] There is also evidence that the globe becomes downwardly displaced owing to loss of support exerting a downward pressure on the orbital fat and outward pressure on the orbital septum. This formed the basis of the approach to return the fat to the orbit by securing the capsulopalpebral fascia to the orbital rim periosteum.[9] The medial and central fat pads are divided by the inferior oblique muscle and accentuate the tear trough or nasojugal groove. The lateral fat pad is responsible for the superior convexity and is separated from the central fat pad by the arcuate expansion (**Fig. 5**). It has been shown that the lower intraorbital fat is actually a continuous body of fat, but it is helpful to visualize this as 3 compartments because this is how it is manipulated surgically. It

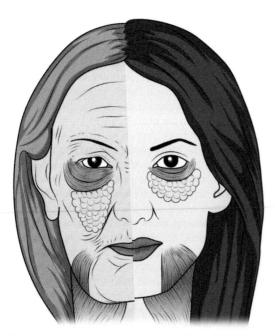

Fig. 1. Aging changes in the lower lid and cheek. In youth, there is a smooth transition from lid to cheek with a full malar mound. With age, the lower lid elongates, the cheek/malar complex descends, and the orbital fat protrudes. All of these changes create a discontinuous double convexity, which is the hallmark of the aging lower lid and cheek. (*From* Buchanan DR, Wulc AE. Contemporary thoughts on lower eyelid/midface aging. Clin Plast Surg 2015;42(1):1–15; with permission.)

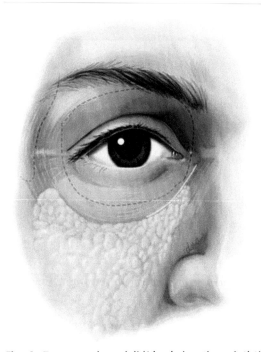

Fig. 3. Tear trough and lid/cheek junction. Artist's drawing depicting the orbicularis oculi muscle junction and the origin of the muscle from the maxilla (*yellow line*). The cleft between the palpebral and orbital portions of the muscle explains the presence of the tear trough (medial) and the lid/cheek junction (lateral). The muscle junction also corresponds precisely to the superior border of the malar fat pad. Note that the orbital rim (*dotted line*) is located several millimeters cephalad to the tear trough and lid/cheek junction. (*From* Haddock NT, Saadeh PB, Boutros S, et al. The tear trough and lid/cheek junction: anatomy and implications for surgical correction. Plast Reconstr Surg 2009;123(4):1336; with permission.)

was posited by Yousif and colleagues[10] that the presence of the inferior oblique muscle medially and the arcuate expansion laterally divide the fat pads by exerting pressure on them as the herniate outward and engulf these structures. In their discussion of the anatomy of the transconjunctival approach, they also describe the presence of the suborbicularis oculi fat (SOOF). With age, the lateral canthal tendon relaxes as well and the lower lid lengthens and the lower lid tarsal support is diminished, thus predisposing to a postoperative lid malposition if unrecognized.

APPROACHES TO LOWER LID REJUVENATION

The earliest blepharoplasties were performed via a transcutaneous approach using either a skin or skin muscle flap through a subciliary incision. In doing so, the pretarsal OOM was violated, causing a loss of support to the tarsus and rounding at the lateral canthus with increased lateral scleral show. The next phase of lower lid rejuvenation involved the excision of orbital fat through a transconjunctival incision, which was described in 1973 by Tessier.[11] In a large study of 400 incisions, this approach has been shown to be safe and effective with few complications.[12] In a comparison of the transconjunctival approach to the transcutaneous approach, there was a 3% rate of permanent scleral show associated with the transconjuctival approach and a 28% rate of permanent scleral show with the transcutaneous approach.[13] Initially, the transconjunctival approach was reserved typically for the younger patient with minimal dermatochalasis and texture change; however, it has gained wide acceptance in periorbital rejuvenation.

Surgeons should be cautious with overresection of the fat because this can produce a hollowed eye that is less youthful and more skeletonized. Moreover, this effect may not manifest itself in the early postoperative period. Manson and colleagues[14] have shown that the globe is moved posteriorly by 2 mm and inferiorly by 1 mm for every 2.5 mL of fat removed.[14] Currently, there is an emphasis on fat conservation with transposition for restoring contour medially and very conservative fat excision in the lateral compartment.

Excess skin is excised conservatively via a skin pinch or skin only flap that is elevated via subciliary incision. This is accompanied usually by a lateral suspension procedure, such as orbicularis suspension. Skin texture changes can also be improved with resurfacing such as laser or chemical peel.

INCISION PLACEMENT

Incision placement for the transconjunctival incision varies from several millimeters below the tarsus to the level of the fornix. A commonly used incision is approximately 8 mm below the lash line or lid margin. Peng and colleagues[15] recommend an incision that is directly overlying the fat as it presents itself when the globe is retropulsed and the lid retracted inferiorly. Closure of the incision is highly surgeon dependent. In a study of 400 transconjunctival incisions, complication rates were low among all incisions, including those that were closed and those that were left unclosed.[12] The subciliary incision should be place approximately 2 mm below the lash line. It is not advisable to go lower than this point because the scar becomes more visible the lower the incision is placed. Incision within a millimeter

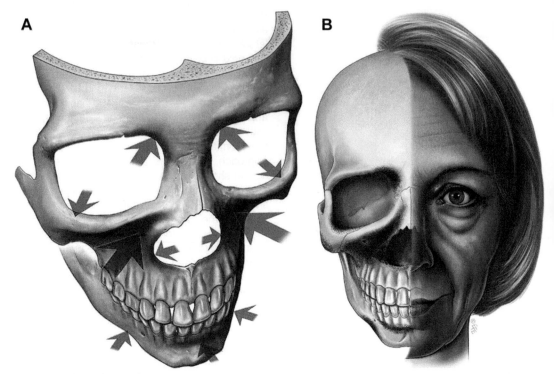

Fig. 4. Facial bone loss with age. Bone loss in the periorbital area and maxilla contributes to the loss of support for the soft tissues and the loss of volume that occurs with age. (*A*) The arrows depict the areas of bone loss and the accompanying changes that occur. (*B*) The stippled areas of the left facial skeleton correspond with the arrows in *A* and the right half of the image depicts the effects this bone loss has on the soft tissues of the face, both in loss of support and volume. (*From* Mendelson B, Wong CH. Anatomy of the aging face. Plastic surgery: volume two. Philadelphia: Elsevier. p. 78–92; with permission.)

of the lashes can result in scarring and distortion of the lash line.

CORRECTION OF THE NASOJUGAL GROOVE (TEAR TROUGH DEFORMITY)

The OOM medially is attached directly to the bone just below the orbital rim (**Box 1, Fig. 6**). The tear trough is created when medial cheek tissues become ptotic and the orbital rim becomes exposed. This is accentuated by pseudoherniated fat from the medial (nasal) and central fat compartments. Correction of this deformity is directed at transposition of the fat or fat/septum inferiorly to fill the defect.[16–19] The nasal and central fat pads are accessed either through a preseptal dissection or a postseptal dissection. Some have posited that the use of the postseptal plane preserves the lower lid retractors (capsulopalpebral fascia) and prevents scarring of the middle lamella (orbital septum) and thus prevents lid malposition. In a study comparing preseptal and postseptal dissections, there was no difference in the incidence of lid malposition and the rate of lid malposition was very low in both groups.[20] Once developed,

the fat pedicle can be transposed subperiosteally or supraperiosteally. The perceived advantage of the subperiosteal pocket is that there is less bleeding and there is a complete release of the tissues. The placement of the skin subperiosteally is thought by some, however, to be less effective in the effacement of the defect as the periosteum is thick and obscures the filling effect of the fat flap. Proponents of supraperiosteal placement of the fat flap argue that there is a more complete effacement of the deformity as the muscle is released from its bony attachments and the supraperiosteal pocket allows for improved expansion of the defect. Supraperiosteal release is associated with more bleeding in this author's experience, but the bleeding is controlled easily with gentle pressure for several minutes. In either case, it is important to develop a complete medial and central flap that is not tethered by the inferior oblique, because this attachment can cause traction on the muscle and can result in transient diplopia or incomplete correction of the nasojugal fold. It is also imperative not to injure the inferior oblique during this process. Comparison of the subperiosteal and supraperiosteal placement

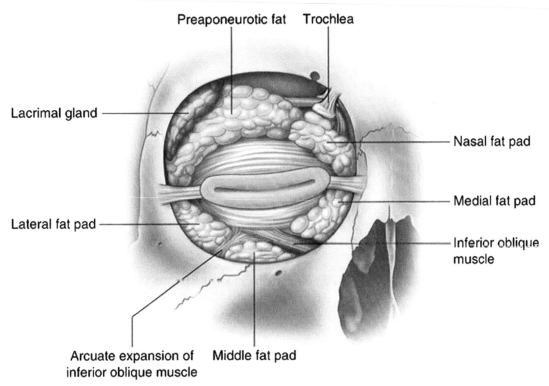

Preaponeurotic fat   Trochlea

Lacrimal gland

Nasal fat pad

Medial fat pad

Lateral fat pad

Inferior oblique muscle

Arcuate expansion of   Middle fat pad
inferior oblique muscle

Fig. 5. Infraorbital fat pads. The medial and central fat pads are divided by the inferior oblique muscle and accentuate the medial tear trough. The lateral fat pad is responsible for the superior convexity laterally and is separated from the central fat pad by the arcuate expansion. It is important not to injure the inferior oblique or arcuate expansion when developing fat pedicles for transposition. (*From* Tan KS, Oh SR, Priel A, et al. Surgical anatomy of the forehead, eyelids, and midface for the aesthetic surgeon. In: Massry GG, Murphy MR, Azizzadeh B, editors. Master techniques in blepharoplasty and periorbital rejuvenation. New York: Springer-USA; 2011. p. 16; with permission.)

of the fat yielded no clinically discernable difference in the effacement of the tear trough with a high degree of patient satisfaction in both groups.[21]

Redundant orbital septum and fat as a composite flap, known as a septal reset, has also been advocated to restore contour to the nasojugal groove.[22] In this procedure, the dissection is

---

Box 1
Steps in correction of the nasojugal groove (tear trough deformity)

1. Location of the tear trough and infraorbital nerve are marked.

2. Transconjunctival incision is made and conjunctival flap is retracted with a stay suture to protect the cornea

3. Dissection inferiorly to the arcus marginalis in the preseptal plane between the orbicularis oculi and the orbital septum. This can alternatively be done in the postseptal plane.

4. Incision of the orbital septum and exposure of the intraorbital fat.

5. Development of the medial and central fat pads. Care should be taken not to injure or tether the inferior oblique muscle. The fat pads should slide freely around the inferior oblique.

6. Blunt dissection of the supraperiosteal pocket to a level below the tear trough. Care is taken not to injure the infraorbital nerve. Bleeding in this area can be controlled with gentle pressure.

7. Fat pads are sutured with a mattress suture on a double armed needle. The medial and central fat pads can be transposed individually or as a unit.

8. The pedicled fat pads are transposed into the pocket and anchored via transcutaneous suture and a bolster. A bolster is left in place for 5 to 7 days.

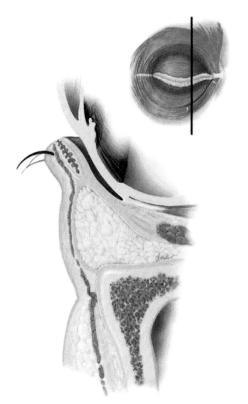

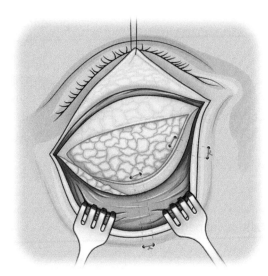

Fig. 7. Septal reset for correction of the nasojugal groove. Redundant orbital septum/fat is transposed as a unit and is sutured through the muscle and skin in a mattress fashion to efface the nasojugal groove. (*From* Pepper JP, Baker S. Transcutaneous lower lid blepharoplasty with fat transposition. Clin Plastic Surg 2015;42(1):60; with permission.)

Fig. 6. Tear trough deformity (nasojugal groove). Medially, the tear trough or nasojugal groove is formed by a direct attachment of the oribicularis oculi muscle just below the orbital rim. Note there is no intervening ligamentous structure as there is in the lateral portion. (*From* Haddock NT, Saadeh PB, Boutros S, et al. The tear trough and lid/cheek junction: anatomy and implications for surgical correction. Plast Reconstr Surg 2009;123(4):1337; with permission.)

preseptal down to the arcus marginalis and the septum in incised widely at this point releasing the fat. The redundant septum and fat are transposed over the orbital rim as a composite flap with anchoring to the periosteum or by fixing it anteriorly with transcutaneous mattress sutures over a bolster to the external skin (**Fig. 7**).

LATERAL SUSPENSION AND CONTOUR CORRECTION

Laterally, the OOM is attached to the bone via the orbital retaining ligament (**Fig. 8**). In this location, the intraorbital fat pad is not transposed over the orbital rim, but rather excised conservatively. Suspension of the lateral tissues helps to efface the transition from lid to cheek. Lateral suspension can take many forms. For those patients who need minimal effacement of the lid/cheek junction and tightening of the lower lid, an orbicularis

suspension of the preseptal orbicularis is effective. The SOOF lift offers a mechanism for restoring contour in the moderately ptotic cheek and the subperiosteal midface lift offers the most aggressive form of correction to this area. The surgeon should use a graded approach to the solution depending on the etiology and severity of the problem.

ORBICULARIS SUSPENSION

The preseptal orbicularis suspension allows for tightening and suspension of the lax or ptotic preseptal orbicularis muscle. When combined with fat excision, this can efface the superior lateral convexity and when combined with a skin only lateral skin excision can provide a mechanism to deal with mild dermatochalasis of the lower lids. This can be accomplished with superolateral suspension of the preseptal orbicularis to the orbital periosteum or the superior limb of the lateral canthal tendon. It may be necessary to try several different target areas of the orbicularis to find the "sweet spot" that will accomplish tightening without distortion. This author prefers to use a braided absorbable suture for this purpose (**Fig. 9**).

SUBORBICULARIS OCULI FAT LIFT

Hwang and associates[23] have shown that the SOOF is concentrated inferolaterally in the

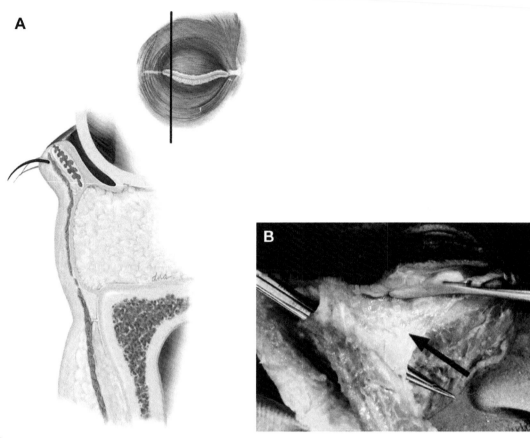

Fig. 8. Orbicularis retaining ligament. (*A*) A sagittal representation of the anatomy of the lateral orbicularis. Laterally, the orbicularis oculi muscle is attached to the bone via the orbicularis retaining ligament (*arrow in B*). This point of attachment corresponds with the groove seen at the lid/cheek junction laterally. (*B*) The orbicularis retaining ligament is dissected (above the scissors) to show its attachment to the orbital periosteum and the orbicularis oculi muscle. This ligament must be lysed to effect movement of the cheek tissues superiorly to efface the lid cheek junction and improve the lateral contour. (*From* Haddock NT, Saadeh PB, Boutros S, et al. The tear trough and lid/cheek junction: anatomy and implications for surgical correction. Plast Reconstr Surg 2009;123(4):1332–40; with permission.)

periorbital tissues in a plane between the orbicularis and the periosteum just at or below the orbital rim. There is a large horizontal portion and a smaller vertical portion that gives this structure a hockey stick appearance[23] (**Fig. 10**). It is a consistent feature of the anatomy of this area and can be used as a means to effect lateral contour correction.[24] Once released, this can be lifted and suspended to the orbital periosteum.[25] As previously mentioned, the orbicularis laterally is connected to the periosteum via the orbicularis retaining ligament. This must be lysed to obtain adequate release and elevation of the tissues.

MIDFACIAL SUBPERIOSTEAL LIFT

Correction of midfacial convexity and ptosis requires midfacial release and resuspension.

Through a lateral extension of a lower lid subciliary incision or via an extension of the upper lid blepharoplasty incision laterally, a subperiosteal pocket can be elevated starting at the arcus marginalis and extending inferiorly to the level of the origin of the masseter on the body of the zygoma.[26] The orbital retaining ligament can be released, allowing the malar mound to be elevated and the midface to be resuspended. Care must be taken with extensive inferolateral dissections not to injure the motor innervation to the orbicularis oculi. A zone approximately 5 mm in diameter located 2.5 cm inferolateral from the lateral canthus represents a critical zone where the nerves are at most risk.[27] Weakness of the OOM is one of several factors predisposing to lid malposition along with eyelid laxity, negative vector eyelid, anterior lamellar shortage, and inferior eyelid/orbital

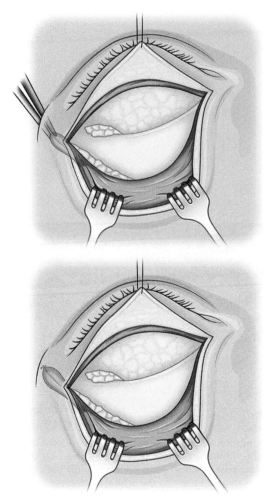

Fig. 9. Orbicularis suspension for lateral contour improvement. A skin only flap is dissected laterally to expose the lateral preseptal orbicularis oculi muscle. This portion of preseptal orbicularis is then suspended to the lateral periosteum of the zygoma. Excess skin is excised conservatively. (*From* Pepper JP, Baker SR. Transcutaneous lower bleparoplasty with fat transposition. Clin Plast Surg 2015;42(1):57–62; with permission.)

volume deficit.[28] For patients with less severe ptosis, a supraperiosteal elevation with SOOF lift can be performed.

AUTOLOGOUS FAT AUGMENTATION

When inadequate fat is present for adequate contour correction, autologous fat can be used to supplement or replace fat transposition as needed.[29] The techniques for periorbital filler and fat injection are discussed elsewhere in this issue and should be kept in mind for use in periorbital rejuvenation in appropriately selected patients (see Chi JJ:

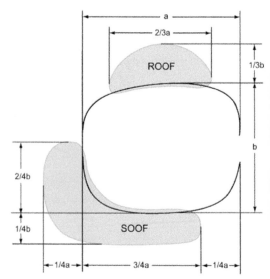

Fig. 10. Dimensions of the suborbicularis oculi fat (SOOF). The SOOF is located inferolaterally to the orbital rim in a hockey stick configuration. The horizontal dimension of the SOOF corresponds with the transverse orbital dimension or approximately 4.8 cm. The vertical dimension is approximately 2.7 cm and corresponds to about three-fourths of the total orbital vertical dimension. ROOF, retroorbicularis oculus fat. (*From* Hwang S, Hwang K, Jin S, et al. Location and nature of retro-orbicularis oculus fat and suborbicularis oculi fat. J Craniofacial Surgery 2007;18(2):389; with permission.)

Periorbital Surgery: Forehead, Brow, and Midface, in this issue; and Glaser DA, Kurta A: Periorbital Rejuvenation: Overview of Non-surgical Treatment Options, in this issue).

DERMATOCHALASIS OF THE LOWER LIDS

The treatment of excessive lower lid skin is dictated by the severity of the problem and by what other procedures are planned as a part of the surgical rejuvenation. Specifically, the degree of elevation of the malar/cheek complex will determine how much redundant skin remains. In all cases, this should be done in a conservative and tension-free manner so that there is no tendency for contraction of the anterior lamella and downward displacement of the lid or frank ectropion. Typically, this is done with a skin pinch or subciliary incision and elevation of a skin only flap. The skin excision is greatest at the lateral canthus and gradually tapers as it progresses medially. Care should be taken to avoid the pretarsal orbicularis and careful preoperative assessment of lid laxity will determine if lateral canthopexy or tarsal strip procedure will be necessary to provide adequate support to the lower lid.

FESTOONS

The presence of festoons or large bags that are typically below the orbital rim and may present as large edematous bags or as a flaccid almost flap like area of excess skin or skin and muscle. Patients may relate that they appear more fluid filled at times and more flat at others. It may be that the repeated inflation/deflation cycle of the tissues that is responsible for the extreme dermatochalasis that develops over time. They can be present in the pretarsal (less common), preseptal, orbital, or malar components of the lid/cheek. Like most of the aging changes that have been discussed, festoons are related to the downward descent of the heavy cheek tissues, the laxity of the orbicularis and orbital retaining ligament, and dermatochalasis of the lower lid skin.[30] Treatment is divided into several categories depending on the assessment of the components of the festoons and their severity and location. Surgical treatment can include a malar or mid-cheek lift with lysis of the orbital retaining ligament, elevation of the SOOF and suspension, which is aimed at correction of the laxity of the orbital retaining ligament and the cheek ptosis. If the festoon is thin and primarily skin or skin and muscle, then direct excision has been used to improve these. In cases of milder festooning, resurfacing with a laser or chemical peel or other device such as a radiofrequency device has been advocated. Patients should be warned, however, that when these festoons are treated with a resurfacing modality, they tend to swell and look worse for quite some time.

SUMMARY

Addressing the contour is essential to rejuvenation of the lower lid. The lower eyelid and malar/cheek complex must be viewed as a single continuous unit. The medial and central fat pads can be used as a fat or fat/septal unit to transpose inferiorly into the tear trough. Lateral fat pads are most often excised conservatively. In many cases, the malar/cheek complex must be released and elevated as well by preseptal orbicularis suspension, SOOF lift or subperiosteal midface lifting. Severity of the aging changes and individual anatomic differences will dictate the appropriate surgical procedure(s) to be performed for successful periorbital lower lid rejuvenation.

REFERENCES

1. Hamra ST. The role of orbital fat preservation in facial aesthetic surgery—a new concept. Clin Plast Surg 1996;23:17–28.
2. Hamra ST. Arcus marginalis release and orbital fat preservation in midface rejuvenation. Plast Reconstr Surg 1995;96:354–62.
3. Nakra T. Biplanar contour-oriented approach to lower eyelid and midface rejuvenation. JAMA Facial Plast Surg 2015;17(5):374–81.
4. Reilly M, Tomsic JA, Fernandez SJ, et al. Effect of facial rejuvenation surgery on perceived attractiveness, femininity, and personality. JAMA Facial Plast Surg 2015;17(3):202–7.
5. Little A, Jones B, DeBruine L. Facial attractiveness: evolutionary based research. Philos Trans R Soc Lond B Biol Sci 2011;366:1638–59.
6. Fezza JP, Massry G. Lower eyelid length. Plast Reconstr Surg 2015;136(2):152e–9e.
7. Pessa JE, Zadoo VP, Mutimer KL, et al. Relative maxillary retrusion as a natural consequence of aging: combining skeletal and soft-tissue changes into an integrated model of midfacial aging. Plast Reconstr Surg 1998;102(1):205–12.
8. Rohrich RJ, Pessa JE. The fat compartments of the face: anatomy and clinical implications for cosmetic surgery. Plast Reconstr Surg 2007;119(7):2219–27.
9. de la Plaza R, Arroyo JM. A new technique for the treatment of palpebral bags. Plast Reconstr Surg 1988;81(5):677–85.
10. Yousif NJ, Sonderman P, Dzwiersynski WW, et al. Anatomic considerations in transconjunctival blepharoplasty. Plast Reconstr Surg 1995;96(6):1271–6.
11. Tessier P. The conjuctival approach to the orbital floor and maxilla in congenital malformation and trauma. J Maxillofac Surg 1973;1(1):3–8.
12. Mullins JB, Holds JB, Branham GH, et al. Complications of the transconjunctival approach. A review of 400 cases. Arch Otolaryngol Head Neck Surg 1997;123(4):385–8.
13. Appling WD, Patrinely JR, Salzer TA. Transconjunctival approach vs subciliary skin-muscle flap approach for orbital fracture repair. Arch Otolaryngol Head Neck Surg 1993;119(9):1000–7.
14. Manson P, Clifford C, Iliff N, et al. Mechanisms of global support and posttraumatic enophthalmos: I. The anatomy of the ligament sling and its relation to the intramuscular cone orbital fat. Plast Reconstr Surg 1986;77:193–202.
15. Peng GL, Jacono A, Massry GG. Globe retropulsion and eyelid depression (GRED)-a surgeon-controlled, unimanual maneuver to access postseptal fat in transconjunctival lower blepharoplasty. Ophthal Plast Reconstr Surg 2014;30(3):273–4.
16. Goldberg RA. The three periorbital hollows: a paradigm for periorbital rejuvenation. Plast Reconstr Surg 2005;116(6):1796–804.
17. Goldberg RA, Edelstein C, Balch K, et al. Fat repositioning in lower eyelid blepharoplasty. Semin Ophthalmol 1998;13(3):103–6.

18. Loeb R. Fat pad sliding and fat grafting for leveling lid depressions. Clin Plast Surg 1981;8:757.

19. Davison SP, Irio M, Oh C. Transconjunctival lower lid blepharoplasty with and without fat repositioning. Clin Plast Surg 2015;42(1):51–6.

20. Schwarcz R, Fezza JP, Jacono A, et al. Stop blaming the septum. Ophthal Plast Reconstr Surg 2015;10(10):1–4.

21. Yoo DB, Peng GL, Massry GG. Transconjuctival lower blepharoplasty with fat repositioning. A retrospective comparison of transposing fat to the subperiosteal vs supraperiosteal planes. JAMA Facial Plast Surg 2013;15(3):176–81.

22. Pepper JP, Baker SR. Transcutaneous lower blepharoplasty with fat transposition. Clin Plast Surg 2015;42(1):57–62.

23. Hwang SH, Hwang K, Jin S, et al. Location and nature of retro-orbicularis oculus fat and suborbicularis oculi fat. J Craniofac Surg 2007;18(2):387–90.

24. Aiache AE, Ramirez OH. The suborbicularis oculi fat pads: an anatomic and clinical study. Plast Reconstr Surg 1995;95(1):37–42.

25. Freeman MS. Transconjunctival Sub–Orbicularis Oculi Fat (SOOF) pad lift blepharoplasty: a new technique for the effacement of nasojugal deformity. Arch Facial Plast Surg 2000;2(1):16–21.

26. Sullivan PK, Drolet BC. Extended lower lid blepharoplasty for eyelid and midface rejuvenation. Plast Reconstr Surg 2013;132(5):1093–101.

27. Hwang K. Surgical anatomy of the lower eyelid relating to lower blepharoplasty. Anat Cell Biol 2010;43(1):15–24.

28. Griffin G, Azizzadeh B, Massry GG. New insights into physical findings associated with postblepharoplasty lower eyelid retraction. Aesthetic Surg J 2014;34(7):995–1004.

29. Einan-Lifshitz A, Holds JB, Wulc AE, et al. Volumetric rejuvenation of the tear trough with repo and Ristow. Ophthal Plast Reconstr Surg 2013;29(6):481–5.

30. Endara M, Oh C, Davison SP, et al. The management of festoons. Clin Plast Surg 2015;42(1):87–94.

Injectable Adjunctive Procedures for Cosmesis and Function

Morris E. Hartstein, MD, FACS

KEYWORDS

• Lid malposition • Ectropion • Retraction • Tear trough • Preperiosteal • Hollow

KEY POINTS

• The role of hyaluronic acid (HA) fillers in the periocular region continues to expand.
• In addition to cosmetic uses in the periocular region, HA fillers are increasingly being used to correct eyelid malpositions.
• This is changing the perspective on the anatomic changes responsible for these malpositions.

Hyaluronic acid (HA) fillers have been in use for many years for cosmetic rejuvenation of the face, specifically for hollows, rhytides, and volume augmentation.[1–5] More recently, however, fillers have been increasingly used as an alternative to traditional surgical procedures. This article discusses various applications in which fillers are being used beyond the usual cosmetic indications in the periocular region.

One of the most popular uses for HA filler in the periocular region is to treat the tear trough. The tear trough, often referred to by patients as dark circles below the eyes, represents a thinning of the tissues and is bounded by the orbitomalar or orbital retaining ligament.[6] Actually, the hollows around the eye include the tear trough, the temporal inferior orbital rim, the center of the cheek where there may be the "V" deformity, and the superior sulcus. However, the tear trough area seems to draw the most attention from patients.

Before the era of fillers, when a patient would present with complaints of lower lid bags, dark circles, or other issues, surgical options were presented that included subtractive blepharoplasty, blepharoplasty with fat repositioning, midface lifting, implants, or any combination of the above. However, fillers offer a nonsurgical alternative in which the bags or dark circles are camouflaged by filling the hollows around them (**Fig. 1**). This technique produces impressive results that can be achieved during a brief office procedure without the downtime associated with surgery.[7–9] Moreover, using fillers instead of traditional subtractive or excisional lifting procedures in the lower lid has advanced knowledge of the aging process so that the role of volume loss is better understood.

When performing filler injections to the tear trough region or the orbital hollows, it is important to remember that this area contains the thinnest skin on the face and is the least forgiving.[10] The injections should be performed in the deep preperiosteal plane. Small aliquots are injected slowly as the needle is withdrawn so as not to raise the hydrostatic pressure. The injection can also be carried with a cannula. Lumps and bumps can be very unsightly and may need to be dissolved with hyaluronidase. Also, not every patient is an ideal candidate for filler treatment in this area. The ideal patient will have a relatively short and shallow tear trough, with minimal to moderate fat prolapse, with minimal skin laxity. A less ideal patient will have significant fat prolapse; a deep and long trough or hollow; and thin, lax skin. Filler in these patients can lead to improvement but results may be suboptimal.

Department of Ophthalmology, Assaf Harofeh Medical Center, Tel Aviv University Sackler School of Medicine, David Elazar 45, Raanana 43204, Israel
E-mail address: mhartstein@earthlink.net

Facial Plast Surg Clin N Am 24 (2016) 139–144
http://dx.doi.org/10.1016/j.fsc.2015.12.005
1064-7406/16/$ – see front matter

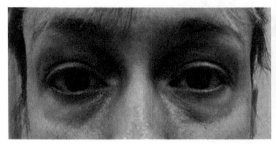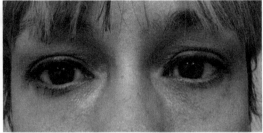

Fig. 1. (*Left*) This woman presented for lower blepharoplasty. (*Right*) After HA filler injection to orbital hollows along the inferior rim. No surgery was performed.

To perform a tear trough, lower lid hollow, injection, follow these guidelines:

- Slow injection
- Stay deep
- Preperiosteal
- Avoid lumps
- Avoid Tyndall

The role of volume augmentation versus lifting has also come into play in the brow region.[11,12] Many procedures for brow lifting have been described, including but not limited to direct brow lift, internal brow lift, temporal subcutaneous brow lift, endoscopic brow lift, and others. However, there is an element of brow deflation as part of the aging process that may be as significant as perceived brow descent. By reinflating the brow using HA fillers and correcting the volume loss that comes with aging, the brow region can often be rejuvenated without the need for surgical lifting procedures. The HA filler is injected beneath the brow, usually in the temporal region. This corrects volume loss, which often occurs in this area, but will also produce some elevation of the brow (**Fig. 2**). This may be used in conjunction with neuromodulators. However, fillers to the brow region may also represent an alternative to neuromodulators because there is less chance of creating a brow contour deformity and it provides a more long-lasting effect.

Another area in which HA fillers are playing an increasingly important role is filling the hollow superior sulcus. Most people have a full superior sulcus when they are young. The orbital rim is not visible and the amount of tarsal platform show is usually minimal.[13] An even cursory glance at the latest fashion magazine will show that beautiful models all demonstrate these features of their upper lids, as opposed to a hollowed out superior sulcus with a large amount of tarsal platform show. With age, however, a hollow superior sulcus can develop. There is baring of the superior orbital rim and increased tarsal platform show.[14] This situation can also occur with overaggressive upper blepharoplasty. For many surgeons, the goal of upper blepharoplasty is to remove all of the perceived excess skin, which may not necessarily produce a more youthful appearance.

Before the HA fillers, when a patient presented with a hollow superior sulcus, treatment options included autologous fat transfer, dermis fat grafting, or possible orbital fat repositioning. With the advent of HA fillers, the hollow superior sulcus can be corrected easily in a quick office procedure.[15–18] When discussing facial rejuvenation, his area is often neglected compared with the lower lid, cheeks, jowls, and neck. By restoring the full lid, eliminating the skeletonization of superior rim, and decreasing tarsal platform show, the aging process is reversed and a youthful appearance restored. This is also an excellent treatment to correct an overaggressive upper blepharoplasty (**Fig. 3**).

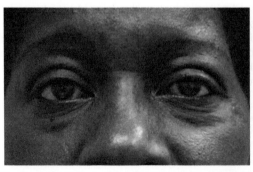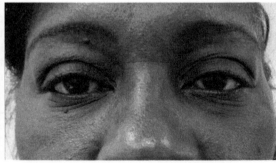

Fig. 2. (*Left*) Patient with left brow ptosis. (*Right*) Following subbrow and tear trough filler injection.

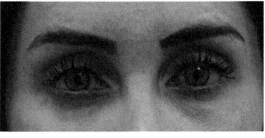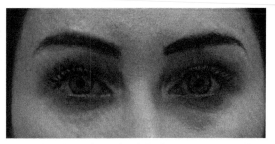

Fig. 3. (*Left*) Patient with hollow superior sulcus following upper blepharoplasty. (*Right*) After correction with HA filler.

To fill the hollow superior sulcus, attempts should not be made to try and fill the hollow directly as is done with other depressions in the face. In the upper lid, this will not be successful and will be like attempting to fill a black hole. Rather, the injections are carried out superficially, starting above the fold, just beneath the brow. Instead of trying to fill a depression, it is helpful to think of this process as unfolding the lid, beginning from the top (**Fig. 4**). The HA filler material is placed superficially in the skin, slowly working inferiorly. At a certain point, the in-folded lid will seem to pop out. At this point additional volume can be given directly into the new fold as needed.

To fill the superior sulcus, follow these guidelines:

- Begin superiorly (beneath the brow)
- Inject superficially
- Work inferiorly
- Wait for lid to seem to pop out
- Add filler to fold as needed

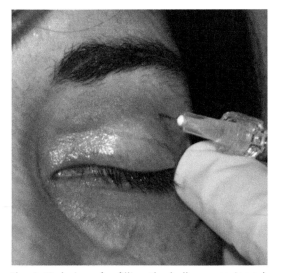

Fig. 4. Technique for filling the hollow superior sulcus. HA filler is injected superficially, above hollow area, progressively injecting more inferiorly.

A similar indication is for patients who have undergone eye removal surgery. Despite placement of spherical implants to replace the eye that is removed, these patients are often left with a very hollow superior sulcus. Before the advent of HA fillers, this deformity would often be corrected surgically by placing subperiosteal implants along the orbital floor or exchanging the spherical implant for a larger one. Obviously, these were significant surgeries to undergo with possible prolonged recovery and the need for prosthesis refit. Now, using HA fillers, the deep superior sulcus can be obliterated during a relatively brief office procedure. The technique is the same as outlined previously, although usually larger amounts of filler material are required.

Patients with seventh nerve palsy often present to the eye specialist with lagophthalmos resulting in dry eye of varying severity. When the exposure is severe, the cornea is in danger of developing an ulcer despite aggressive lubrication. Surgical intervention includes tarsorrhaphy, which allows the cornea to heal but which most patients find extremely unsightly and uncomfortable. Another treatment is a gold weight implant placed in the upper lid to achieve full closure when a blink is initiated. However, gold weights, being foreign bodies, can cause allergic reactions or extrude (**Fig. 5**). With HA fillers, it is possible to create a lid load in the same way as a gold weight.[19] However, with HA fillers, the amount of load can be titrated according to patient need. The injection is performed in similar fashion to the superior sulcus (**Fig. 6**). For the patient in the intensive care unit, this is an easy bedside procedure that can save the cornea.

One of the most exciting new applications for HA fillers is the correction of lower eyelid malposition, ectropion, or lid retraction.[20,21] This may be involutional as a result of lid laxity or may result from an overly aggressive lower lid blepharoplasty. These retracted lower lids are often difficult and challenging to correct. Surgery may involve a lateral canthoplasty, placement of a spacer graft,

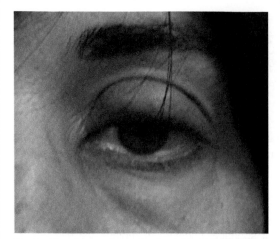

Fig. 5. Allergic reaction to implanted gold weight left upper lid for paralytic lagophthalmos.

midface lift, and frost sutures to put the lid on stretch for up to 7 days. Horizontal lid tightening plays an important role in the correction of ectropion or retraction; however, there is another component as well. The analogy of a hammock is often used regarding the lower lid. Tightening the hammock (ie, horizontal lid tightening) will help raise the lid. However, we can also picture the ectropion lid as in-folded similar to in the hollow upper lid. Therefore, filler may be used to unfold the lower lid and provide greater support from below for the hammock.

Another component of lower lid malposition is the negative vector. A negative vector is found when the eye-globe protrudes more anteriorly than the lid and cheek tissues inferiorly. A negative vector predisposes the lid to become retracted, especially after blepharoplasty surgery. Some postblepharoplasty lid retraction patients may have had an unrecognized negative vector preoperatively, which likely played a role in the development of the lid malposition. However,

some patients are left with a negative vector after overaggressive removal of lower eyelid tissue during blepharoplasty. In these patients, even the combination of surgical procedures previously described will have difficulty yielding a successful result due to the negative vector because the lid needs to be advanced anteriorly as well as lifted vertically. Again, this is another place in which injectable HA fillers can play an important role. By using fillers in the lower lid, the negative vector can at least be decreased and sometimes even eliminated. The filling procedure alone may result in correction of the lid position. If there is still residual retraction following filler injection, it can still enable easier surgical correction because the negative vector does not need to be overcome with surgery. Now the lid just needs be lifted vertically.

When injecting HA fillers to correct lower lid retraction, the injections are begun inferiorly along the orbital rim and deep in the preperiosteal space. Gradually, the injections are carried out more superiorly and more superficially toward the lid margin. As the lid is unfolded, it is also advanced superiorly (**Figs. 7** and **8**). In cases in which the lower lid is tethered to the orbital rim from fibrotic tissue, filler injection is unlikely to overcome this.

To correct lower lid malposition, follow these guidelines:

- Inject slowly
- Stay deep
- Begin at inferior rim
- Work superiorly toward lid margin
- Inject superficially at lid margin

Complications can occur from HA fillers in the periocular region as in other areas of the face.[22–26] Because of the thin eyelid skin, there may be more chance of visible lumps and the so-called Tyndall effect in this region. If an unsightly lump does occur, it can be dissolved with hyaluronidase but often that will mean starting all over again.

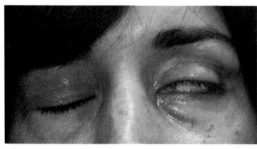
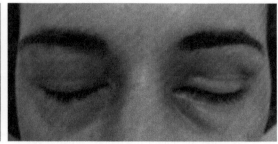

Fig. 6. (*Left*) Left lagophthalmos secondary to seventh nerve palsy with corneal exposure. (*Right*) HA filler used to load left upper lid until no lagophthalmos remains.

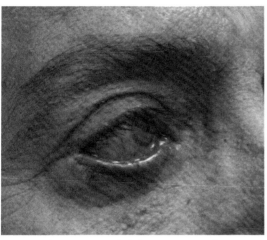 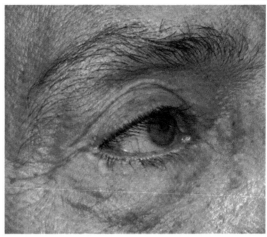

Fig. 7. (*Left*) Patient with lid retraction and ectropion following glower blepharoplasty and one attempted repair. (*Right*) Complete correction of lid malposition with HA filler only to unfold, raise, and reappose the lower lid to the globe.

Thus, it is advised to proceed slowly, possibly in stages, when using filler in the periocular region. Vascular occlusion affecting vision can occur from injections elsewhere on the face. However, when injecting, for example, in the superior sulcus, this is in very close proximity to the supraorbital vessels and thus extreme care should be used.

This article demonstrates the role of HA fillers for correction of eyelid malpositions and deformities that were previously considered to be surgical procedures. More than just providing an easier and quicker alternative to surgery, the use of HA fillers in the periocular region has enhanced understanding of the aging changes taking place. Whereas the focus used to be on correcting descent of soft tissues, now much more emphasis is placed on correcting deflation of the soft tissues. Lid malpositions can often be corrected by simply replacing volume, avoiding the need for surgical lifting and tightening procedures.

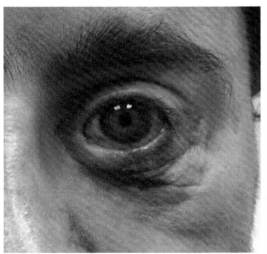 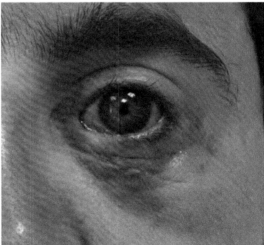

Fig. 8. (*Left*) Patient with left lower lid retraction secondary to Mobius syndrome, after several surgical attempts at repair, including midface lift. (*Right*) Following correction of lid retraction with filler only to unfold and elevate lid to inferior limbus.

REFERENCES

1. Pao KY, Mancini R. Nonsurgical periocular rejuvenation: advanced cosmetic uses of neuromodulators and fillers. Curr Opin Ophthalmol 2014;25(5):461–9.
2. Pavicic T, Few JW, Huber-Vorländer J. A novel, multi-step, combination facial rejuvenation procedure for treatment of the whole face with incobotulinumtoxinA, and two dermal fillers- calcium hydroxylapatite and a monophasic, polydensified hyaluronic acid filler. J Drugs Dermatol 2013;12(9):978–84.
3. Callan P, Goodman GJ, Carlisle I, et al. Efficacy and safety of a hyaluronic acid filler in subjects treated for correction of midface volume deficiency: a 24 month study. Clin Cosmet Investig Dermatol 2013; 6:81–9.
4. Tung R, Ruiz de Luzuriaga AM, Park K, et al. Brighter eyes: combined upper cheek and tear trough augmentation: a systematic approach utilizing two complementary hyaluronic acid fillers. J Drugs Dermatol 2012;11(9):1094–7.
5. Muhn C, Rosen N, Solish N, et al. The evolving role of hyaluronic acid fillers for facial volume restoration and contouring: a Canadian overview. Clin Cosmet Investig Dermatol 2012;5:147–58.
6. Wong CH, Hsieh MK, Mendelson B. The tear trough ligament: anatomical basis for the tear trough deformity. Plast Reconstr Surg 2012;129(6):1392–402.
7. Goldberg RA, Fiaschetti D. Filling the periorbital hollows with hyaluronic acid gel: initial experience with 244 injections. Ophthal Plast Reconstr Surg 2006; 22(5):335–41 [discussion: 341–3].
8. Goldberg RA. Nonsurgical filling of the periorbital hollows. Aesthet Surg J 2006;26(1):69–71.
9. Sharad J. Dermal fillers for the treatment of tear trough deformity: a review of anatomy, treatment techniques, and their outcomes. J Cutan Aesthet Surg 2012;5(4):229–38.
10. Rootman DB, Lin JL, Goldberg R. Does the Tyndall effect describe the blue hue periodically observed in subdermal hyaluronic acid gel placement? Ophthal Plast Reconstr Surg 2014;30(6):524–7.
11. Buckingham ED, Glasgold R, Kontis T, et al. Volume rejuvenation of the facial upper third. Facial Plast Surg 2015;31(1):43–54.
12. Kane MA. Nonsurgical periorbital and brow rejuvenation. Plast Reconstr Surg 2015;135(1):63–71.
13. Glasgold RA, Glasgold MJ, Gerth DJ. Upper eyelid volumization with hyaluronic acid. In: Hartstein ME, Holds JB, Massry GG, editors. Pearls and pitfalls in cosmetic oculoplastic surgery. New York: Springer; 2015. p. 511–8.
14. Papageorgiou KI, Ang M, Chang SH, et al. Aesthetic considerations in upper eyelid retraction surgery. Ophthal Plast Reconstr Surg 2012;28(6):419–23.
15. Hartstein ME. Correcting the upper eyelid hollow with filler. In: Hartstein ME, Holds JB, Massry GG, editors. Pearls and pitfalls in cosmetic oculoplastic surgery. New York: Springer; 2015. p. 519–20.
16. Morley AM, Taban M, Malhotra R, et al. Use of hyaluronic acid gel for upper eyelid filling and contouring. Ophthal Plast Reconstr Surg 2009;25(6):440–4.
17. Mancini R, Khadavi NM, Goldberg RA. Nonsurgical management of upper eyelid margin asymmetry using hyaluronic acid gel filler. Ophthal Plast Reconstr Surg 2011;27(1):1–3.
18. Liew S, Nguyen DQ. Nonsurgical volumetric upper periorbital rejuvenation: a plastic surgeon's perspective. Aesthetic Plast Surg 2011;35(3): 319–25.
19. Mancini R, Taban M, Lowinger A, et al. Use of hyaluronic acid gel in the management of paralytic lagophthalmos: the hyaluronic acid gel "gold weight". Ophthal Plast Reconstr Surg 2009;25(1): 23–6.
20. Fezza JP. Nonsurgical treatment of cicatricial ectropion with hyaluronic acid filler. Plast Reconstr Surg 2008;121(3):1009–14.
21. Goldberg RA, Lee S, Jayasundera T, et al. Treatment of lower eyelid retraction by expansion of the lower eyelid with hyaluronic acid gel. Ophthal Plast Reconstr Surg 2007;23(5):343–8.
22. Carle MV, Roe R, Novack R, et al. Cosmetic facial fillers and severe vision loss. JAMA Ophthalmol 2014;132(5):637–9.
23. Cavallini M, Gazzola R, Metalla M, et al. The role of hyaluronidase in the treatment of complications from hyaluronic acid dermal fillers. Aesthet Surg J 2013;33(8):1167–74.
24. DeLorenzi C. Complications of injectable fillers, part I. Aesthet Surg J 2013;33(4):561–75.
25. Kassir R, Kolluru A, Kassir M. Extensive necrosis after injection of hyaluronic acid filler: case report and review of the literature. J Cosmet Dermatol 2011; 10(3):224–31.
26. Cohen JL, Biesman BS, Dayan SH, et al. Treatment of hyaluronic acid filler-induced impending necrosis with hyaluronidase: consensus recommendations. Aesthet Surg J 2015;35(7):844–9.

Periorbital Rejuvenation
Overview of Nonsurgical Treatment Options

 CrossMark

Dee Anna Glaser, MD*, Anastasia Kurta, DO

KEYWORDS

- Periorbital rejuvenation • Noninvasive • Laser • Chemical peels • Neuromodulators

KEY POINTS

- Aging of the periorbital facial subunit can be improved via topical therapies, mechanical and chemical skin resurfacing techniques, use of lasers and radiofrequency devices, fillers, and neuromodulation by use of botulinum toxin.
- Improvement of skin texture, color, scarring, and wrinkling is an important part of periorbital rejuvenation and can be achieved through many different techniques, including chemical peels, dermabrasion, and laser therapy.
- Neuromodulator use for periocular rejuvenation most commonly targets the glabella lines, brow elevation, brow reshaping, and lateral canthal lines.
- Fillers in the periorbital region can be a great adjunct to other procedures.

INTRODUCTION

The periorbital facial subunit consists of the eyebrows, upper and lower eyelids, glabellar region, and pericanthal area. It is one of the first regions to reveal signs of aging and plays an important role in overall facial appearance. The aging process is influenced by our genetic composition as well as environmental factors. Aging skin is characterized by the appearance of fine and coarse rhytides (wrinkles), rough and uneven texture, dryness, and changes in pigmentation.[1] Animation lines in the glabella and lateral canthi, along with volume loss, add to the aging appearance. Repeated facial expressions, ultraviolet radiation exposure, and cigarette smoking all contribute to decreased skin elasticity and development of aging characteristics. With new advancements in cosmetic medicine, nonsurgical and minimally invasive procedures have become first-line treatment options. Treatments that are commonly used today include topical therapies, mechanical and chemical skin resurfacing techniques, use of lasers and radiofrequency devices, fillers, and neuromodulation by use of botulinum toxin (BoNT). Each of these treatment options provide specific benefits as well as different side-effect profiles and can be combined to maximize results.

TOPICAL THERAPIES

Adjunctive skin care is important in the overall rejuvenation and to help maintain results with other procedures. Given that there are thousands of products available and the high acceptance by patients, it is important that physicians review which products may actually be of value for the patient (**Box 1**). Eyelid skin is the thinnest in the body and can be sensitive to any of the topical products.[2]

Department of Dermatology, Saint Louis University School of Medicine, 1755 South Grand Boulevard, St Louis, MO 63104, USA
* Corresponding author.
E-mail address: glasermd@slu.edu

Facial Plast Surg Clin N Am 24 (2016) 145–152
http://dx.doi.org/10.1016/j.fsc.2016.01.003
1064-7406/16/$ – see front matter © 2016 Elsevier Inc. All rights reserved.

Box 1
Topicals for periocular rejuvenation

Sunscreens with UVA and UVB protection

Antioxidants

- Vitamin C
- Vitamin E
- Green tea
- Niacinamide

Retinoids

Peptides

Growth factors

Bimatoprost

Sunscreens are indispensable to help prevent photodamage and to help reduce the development of after-procedure hyperpigmentation. To maximize their benefit, a sun protection factor of 30 or higher (for ultraviolet B [UVB] protection) and a "broad spectrum" (for ultraviolet A [UVA] protection) sunscreen should be worn on a daily basis. Many makeup lines will have UVB protection but usually lack adequate UVA protection.

Antioxidants scavenge free radicals, which are capable of damaging cellular membranes, DNA, and proteins within cells. The most commonly used in topical therapies include vitamin C and vitamin E, and combinations of the 2 have been shown to provide more potent photoprotection than either agent alone. Niacinamide has anti-inflammatory properties as well and may improve hyperpigmentation by decreasing the transfer of melanosomes to keratinocytes.

The use of topical retinoids improves wrinkles by increasing dermal collagen synthesis and inhibiting dermal collagen degradation. Dyschromia can be improved via inhibition of tyrosinase activity, decreasing melanosome transfer and increasing shedding of keratinocytes. Only tretinoin and tazarotene have US Food and Drug Administration (FDA) approval for the treatment of photodamage, and both can have side effects, such as dryness, redness, flaking, and irritation to the skin, limiting their use by patients. Over-the-counter retinoids such as retinol is less irritating than retinoic acid but is also 20-fold less potent than tretinoin.[2]

Peptides and growth factors are thought to improve wrinkles and lines by upregulating collagen production, downregulating collagen degradation, aiding in tissue repair, and via intercellular signaling. There has been some concern that the use of cosmeceuticals containing human growth factors could be associated with the development of skin cancer in predisposed individuals, although there are no reports in the literature.

Topical bimatoprost 0.03% was FDA-approved in 2008 for the enhancement of eyelashes. Its use results in darkening, increased eyelash length, and density (thickening). Its safety and efficacy have been well established along with a good tolerability profile. The authors have patients apply nightly for 4 months to achieve optimal results; then patients can begin a maintenance regimen of applying the product 3 to 4 nights weekly. In addition, patients can apply the product to the eyebrows, but this is off-label and not well-studied. The most common side effects are redness and pruritus.

It is the practice of the authors to maximize the use of tretinoin and sunscreen before adding other topical agents to their regimen. Gentle cleansers and moisturizers are typically needed to combat the side effects of the tretinoin.

SKIN RESURFACING

Improvement of skin texture, color, scarring, and wrinkling is an important part of periorbital rejuvenation and can be achieved through many different techniques, including chemical peels, dermabrasion, and laser therapy. In general, as the depth of injury increases, the results become more dramatic, but the healing time and potential risks also increase, regardless of the tool or device used. Eye protection is important when performing periocular procedures. Resurfacing can be performed as monotherapy, but more often is used as an adjunct to other therapies and surgical procedures.

CHEMICAL SKIN RESURFACING (PEELS)

Chemical peels are an effective option to treat photodamaged skin, rhytides, scarring, and dyschromia. Based on the depth or level of injury, peels are classified as superficial, medium, or deep.[3] Peels can induce exfoliation, epidermal thickening, skin lightening, and new collagen formation, leading to skin rejuvenation.[4] They have a well-known safety profile, relatively low cost, and predictable downtime.[1] It is particularly important to evaluate the patients' expectations as well as their skin type in order to achieve desired results. Patients with Fitzpatrick skin types IV to VI have increased risk for developing dyspigmentation after treatment as well as hypertrophic and keloid scarring.[4] As a result, these individuals would benefit most from superficial or medium-depth peels. Skin preparation is commonly used before a peel and can include topical tretinoin, hydroquinoine, sun protection, and herpes prophylaxis for deeper peels. The depth of any peel can be altered by the skin preparation, and the method of application of the peeling agent.

Superficial chemical peels affect mainly the epidermis, with occasional involvement of the papillary dermis, and can be used to treat mild acne scarring, mild photoaging, solar lentigenes and keratoses, as well as epidermal dyschromia.[5] The major advantage is that they can be used in all skin types with minimal risk of inducing postinflammatory hyperpigmentation. The types of peels in this category include glycolic acid, salicylic acid, 10% to 25% trichloroacetic acid (TCA), and Jessner solution (combination of resorcinol, salicylic acid, and lactic acid in 95% ethanol) and mainly affect the superficial epidermis.[3] Higher concentrations of glycolic acid (70%) or TCA (25%) can cause the level of injury to extend to the basal layer and create regeneration of the entire epidermis, significantly aiding in the treatment of acne, mild photoaging, and melasma, but not quite as effective to induce dermal remodeling.[3] The depth of the wound caused by the various dilutions of TCA is paramount to the therapeutic efficacy.[6] The side effects of superficial peels are fairly minimal and include irritation, erythema, allergic or contact dermatitis, and temporary burning and stinging sensation. The downside is that repeat series of treatments are generally needed to obtain effective results and are usually separated by several weeks.[4]

Medium-depth chemical peels affect the papillary dermis and part of the upper reticular dermis and can be used for mild to moderate photoaging, mild rhytides, and blending of skin after using other resurfacing procedures.[3] In order to create controlled injury, the agents most commonly used are 35% TCA in combination with Jessner solution, glycolic acid at 70% concentration, or solid carbon dioxide. The depth of injury is determined by the degree of skin frosting, rated from I to III after the acids have been applied (**Table 1**). The Jessner–TCA combination induces new collagen production that persists at least 4 months

after a single treatment and reduces dyschromias due to superficial melanin retention or deposition.[5] Medium-depth peels are especially effective in improving advanced photoaging in the periorbital area. Special care around the eyes is necessary to prevent acid to be wicked into the eye from tearing or into tears running down the cheek, which can cause the peel to travel down the cheek, creating linear streaks.[1] Applying a small amount of petroleum ointment at the lateral canthus can help to prevent these side effects. The expected after-procedure effects include edema, crusting of the skin, and eventually re-epithelization by 1 to 2 weeks.[6]

Deep chemical peels result in tissue injury that affects the midreticular dermis and can be used to improve deeper rhytides, moderate to severe photoaging, and extensive actinic keratoses. The peels in this category include 50% TCA, occluded phenol, and occluded or unoccluded Baker-Gordon formula (3 mL of 88% phenol, 2 mL of tap water, 8 drops of Septisol, and 3 drops of croton oil).[1] Because of the thin skin in the periorbital area, if a deep chemical peel is chosen, a modified Baker-Gordon formula should be used, which includes mineral oil in place of water and fewer drops of croton oil.[1] Deep chemical peels can be very effective, but are also associated with more potential complications, including risk of scarring, textural changes, hyperpigmentation or hypopigmentation, and risk of ectropion of the lower eyelid if used near the eyes. If an ectropion does develop, it tends to be self-limiting and corrects spontaneously or with conservative care.[7] More specifically, phenol peels can cause cardiac, renal, and pulmonary toxicities and require careful cardiac monitoring and hydration with intravenous fluids before and during the procedure to facilitate phenol excretion.[7] Wound-healing process is similar to when medium-depth peels are used, but wound dressings and wound care are necessary due to more extensive dermal damage.

MECHANICAL SKIN RESURFACING (DERMABRASION)

Dermabrasion is a mechanical method of resurfacing skin and includes microdermabrasion, manual dermabrasion, and motorized dermabrasion.[1] Dermabrasion in the periorbital region has declined in popularity with the availability of newer technology, but can still be used to improve skin texture and dyschromia. Microdermabrasion targets the most superficial layer of the skin using a motorized device that rapidly fires and recaptures aluminum oxide or other crystals, or a crystal-free diamond-tipped wand for the

Table 1 Medium depth chemical peel frosting level helps to determine the depth of the peel	
Skin Frosting Rating	**Cutaneous Findings**
I	Erythema with white speckling
II	Predominate white speckling but can still see erythema
III	Solid whitening of skin

removal of skin up to the superficial spinous layer.[8] This particular technique is effective in smoothing the skin texture and reducing dyschromia. It is also advantageous due to virtually no downtime. Typically, these are performed on a regular schedule: monthly to quarterly.

Manual dermabrasion is the most effective of the 3 methods, specifically for use on the eyelids, because it provides greater control in the depth of injury. Manual dermabrasion uses silicon carbide sandpaper, and by variation in the force and duration, as well as number of passes, this procedure can improve deeper rhytides and scars.[8]

Last, motorized dermabrasion uses a wire brush or diamond fraise that is driven by a rotary power motor and is well suited for very deep rhytides because it removes the epidermis and the upper layer of the dermis.[1] Motorized dermabrasion is generally not a good option for the periorbital region because of the technical challenges of the thin and mobile skin of the eyelids. It is quite helpful to improve scars that may be present from direct brow lifts or excision of lesions away from the lids.

LASER RESURFACING (ABLATIVE, NONABLATIVE, AND FRACTIONAL DEVICES) AND RADIOFREQUENCY TECHNOLOGY

Lasers remain one of the most popular methods for skin resurfacing because of their ability to selectively target specific components of the skin at precise depths. Ablative and nonablative laser resurfacing may be used to achieve skin rejuvenation, and generally, ablative lasers produce greater clinical results, but with a higher side-effect profile.[9] Ablative lasers include carbon dioxide (CO_2) and Erbium:Yttrium-Aluminum-Garnet (Er:YAG) laser. These lasers cause destruction of the epidermis and part of the dermis, leading to remodeling of tissue by way of wound healing. Conventionally, full-face resurfacing is recommended to avoid formation of demarcation lines; however, the lower eyelid is an exception and can be treated alone with minimal risk of demarcation.[1]

Carbon Dioxide Laser

Historically, ablative CO_2 laser has been the gold standard for skin resurfacing.[10] At 10,600-nm wavelength, CO_2 lasers target water. All water in tissues absorbs this wavelength of light, which leads to vaporization of the tissue, heat-induced collagen contraction and skin-tightening, hemostasis by thermal injury and coagulation, and eventually, fibroplasia and neocollagen deposition.[1] Patients can obtain significant results after carbon dioxide laser resurfacing especially in the periorbital area.[10] Downsides include prolonged erythema, risk of scarring, hypopigmentation, and lower lid ectropion formation. Specifically, patients with a history of previous blepharoplasty have a higher risk of developing ectropion, and laser parameters must be adjusted accordingly.[11]

Erbium:Yttrium-Aluminum-Garnet Laser

The ablative Er:YAG laser emits light at 2910 nm wavelength; water-containing tissues can be vaporized, similar to the carbon dioxide laser system. In contrast to CO_2 resurfacing, the depth of tissue penetrance is less with the Er:YAG laser and less heat is produced. In a comparative trial, both CO_2 and Er:YAG laser produced similar skin tightening results; however, some physicians reserve it for superficial rhytides, while using a CO_2 laser alone or in combination with the Er:YAG laser for deeper rhytides.[12,13] Specifically, in the periorbital region, however, clinical studies have shown the Er:YAG laser to be effective for both superficial and deep rhytides, likely due to the thinner skin in this region.[14] Er:YAG lasers may produce decreased intensity and duration of erythema, faster recovery time, and decreased risk of scarring, all of which are primarily related to the more shallow ablation. Some of the disadvantages include increased risk of dermal bleeding due to reduced hemostatic effect of the Er:YAG laser, which can impair visibility during treatment, and lack of immediate collagen contracture.[1]

Nonablative and Radiofrequency Devices

Nonablative lasers have become a good treatment option for many patients who are not comfortable with the side-effect profile and longer downtime associated with ablative laser resurfacing. Lasers in this category include midinfrared lasers that target the dermis, visible light lasers such as the 585-nm pulsed dye laser, and the 532-nm pulsed potassium titanyl phosphate laser, the infrared 1450-nm diode laser, and the 1320-nm Nd:YAG laser, among others.[15] Nonablative skin resurfacing produces dermal thermal injury while preserving the epidermis.[15] A major benefit of nonablative lasers is their excellent safety profile with the most common side effects being transient purpura or pigmentary changes.[1] Because the epidermis is left intact, makeup can be worn immediately. These lasers can also be used to treat benign lesions such as sebaceous gland hyperplasia and intradermal nevi.

Radiofrequency resurfacing devices deliver energy to the skin, creating heat in the dermal layer and stimulating collagen formation. The cosmetic effects obtained are similar to nonablative laser resurfacing; however, with radiofrequency devices, the collagen denatures immediately, causing skin contraction, and allows for more immediate results in improving superficial rhytides.[16] Advantages also include lack of significant erythema that resolves within hours and has minimal risk of side effects.[15]

Fractional Laser Resurfacing

Fractional laser resurfacing delivers thermal injury to microscopic columns of tissue in regularly spaced arrays, leaving parts of untreated skin intact, which allows for rapid epithelialization. Fractionated lasers include nonablative and ablative devices. The former creates microscopic columns of thermal injury, sparing the epidermis.[17] There is generally less melanin absorption, which allows successful treatment of higher Fitzpatrick skin types (types IV–VI) and less risk of dyschromia.[17] With nonablative fractional laser treatments, patients often experience mild erythema, which resolves within a week, and mild swelling that resolves in a few days, creating minimal downtime. Several treatment sessions are usually required, spaced about 1 month apart. Despite the typical downtime with the treatment, some patients may exhibit significant periorbital swelling, lasting 2 to 3 days (**Fig. 1**).

Ablative CO_2 fractional laser delivers thermal injury to microscopic columns of epidermal and dermal tissue.[17] The fractionated technology allows the operator to deliver thermal tissue injury and dermal coagulation to greater depths than with traditional CO_2 resurfacing, and as a result, may create greater tissue contraction, collagen production, and dermal remodeling than that seen with nonablative devices.[9] The side effects are also minimized, and in particular, hypopigmentation occurs significantly less with the fractionated technology when compared with the standard ablative approach, avoiding lines of demarcation between the treated and untreated areas.[15] Patients should still be counseled on the risks and careful monitoring for prolonged erythema or delayed wound healing as well as potential for scarring (**Fig. 2**). Overall, clinical results obtained with ablative fractional laser resurfacing are comparative to standard ablative CO_2 resurfacing but with a quicker recovery time and better risk profile. However, more than one treatment may be necessary to optimize outcomes. Similar to traditional CO_2 resurfacing, benefits may take 6 months to be fully realized.

NEUROMODULATION

BoNT has been used since the 1980s to treat strabismus and blepharospasm and in the last 20 years has become the most common cosmetic procedure for facial enhancement. Injection techniques have been well-studied in the periorbital region, and patient satisfaction is very high.[18] BoNT is a naturally occurring heterodimeric neuromodulatory polypeptide, produced by *Clostridium botulinum*.[1] It inhibits acetylcholine release at the neuromuscular junction, reducing muscle contraction. It is taken up in the presynaptic terminal via receptor-mediated endocytosis, and in the acidic environment of the endosome, a disulfide bond breaks, separating the core protein into heavy and light chains.[18] The light chain then cleaves specific proteins; BoNT type A targets SNAP-25 (synaptosomal-associated protein, 25 kDa), while type B cleaves VAMP (vehicle associated

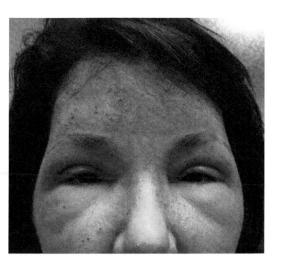

Fig. 1. Significant periorbital edema following fractionated nonablative laser resurfacing.

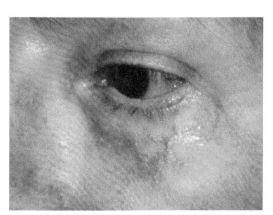

Fig. 2. Early scarring present at lower-eyelid 4 months after fractionated CO_2 laser resurfacing.

membrane protein), leading to blockade of acetylcholine release.[18]

The effects of BoNT are irreversible, but efficacy declines in about 3 to 6 months because of generation of new axon terminals.[18] Before treatment, appropriate patient selection, education, and counseling are crucial. Neuromuscular toxins should not be used in patients who are pregnant (BoNT is category C) or have myasthenia gravis, Eaton-Lambert syndrome, or amyotrophic lateral sclerosis. The most common side effects of BoNT are after-injection erythema, pain, bruising, and headache.[1] A rare side effect in the periorbital region is eyebrow and eyelid ptosis, because of paralysis of the inferior frontalis muscle and levator palpebrae, respectively.[18]

There are currently 4 neurotoxin formulations available for injection in the United States: onabotulinumtoxinA (Botox; Allergan, Inc, Irvine, CA), abobotulinumtoxinA (Dysport; Galderma Laboratories, LP, Fort Worth, TX), incobotulinumtoxinA (Xeomin; Merz Pharmaceuticals, LLC, Greensboro, NC), and rimabotulinumtoxinB (Myobloc; Solstice Neurosciences, Inc, San Francisco, CA).[18] There is significant variation in the concentration of BoNT used by clinicians. Generally, higher concentrations with lower volumes may decrease diffusion as well as pain associated with the injection.[1] Alternatively, lower concentrations may be used in larger muscles such as the frontalis, to increase diffusion.[1]

Neuromodulator use for periocular rejuvenation most commonly targets the glabella lines, brow elevation, brow reshaping, and lateral canthal lines. In addition, the lower eyelids can be treated to open up the palpebral aperture by injecting at the midpupillary line, 2 to 3 mm below the lower eyelid margin. This area should be avoided in patients with significant lower lid laxity because of the risk of potentially worsening the laxity. Forehead injections can also be used but increase the risks of brow ptosis, especially if the injections

are placed in the inferior frontalis muscle or if there is pre-existing brow ptosis. Just as concentrations of BoNT vary, so do the numbers of units (**Table 2**) and numbers of injections. Achieving optimal outcomes for each patient involves a thorough understanding of the anatomy and the patient's desired look. Lower doses will allow for more natural movement in the treated area, but frequently lends to a shorter duration of effect, while higher dosing may give a longer duration but increases the risk of a more "frozen" appearance.[19]

There are many in-depth books and papers on the use of BoNT,[18] but some key tips for periocular injection include the following:

- Look for asymmetries before injection (**Fig. 3**)
- Document with good photographs at rest and with muscle contraction
- Patients frequently are not aware of asymmetries and should be counseled on realistic expectations in terms of achieving symmetry
- Document injection dosing and pattern precisely to assist with future adjustments
- Cheek movement can contribute to the appearance of lateral canthal lines and may be difficult to eradicate with BoNT alone (**Fig. 4**)

In addition, BoNT use before resurfacing has been shown to improve the outcomes of laser resurfacing. Injections are performed 1 to 2 weeks before resurfacing.[20]

FILLERS

Volume loss is a natural phenomenon of the aging process and can be augmented with the use of fillers. It is also a great option for correcting static rhytides that cannot be treated with BoNT alone and to recontour. Hyaluronic acid (HA) is probably the workhorse for the periorbital area because of its good efficacy and predictability, but autologous fat is also very useful for larger volume deficits.[1]

Table 2		
Typical doses of neuromodulator use for periocular rejuvenation		
	OnabotbulinumtoxinA and IncobotulinumtoxinA Units	AbobotulinumtoxinA Units
Glabella frown lines	15–30	40–60
Glabella lines with brow lift bilateral or reshaping	20–35	50–80
Lateral canthal lines bilateral	20–30	40–70
Forehead lines	10–20	20–50
Infraorbital bilateral	2–5	5–15

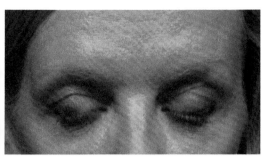

Fig. 3. Baseline eyebrow asymmetry noted at consult for neuromodulator use.

Side effects of using fillers include bruising, erythema, tenderness, and edema. More rarely, injection site necrosis, and arterial embolization and occlusion of the ophthalmic artery, can occur, creating serious complications such as permanent blindness.[1] In addition, depending on the filler compound, hypersensitivity reactions, granuloma formation, uneven distribution, and infections can occur.

HA creates effective cosmetic results, good duration, and minimal complications. This glycosaminoglycan disaccharide consists of alternating units of D-glucouronic acid and N-acetyl-D-glucosamine that are normally present throughout the human tissue, including the skin, synovial joint fluid, and vitreous.[21] Its chemical structure is uniform across species, and among the different commercially available HA fillers, although each final product has unique characteristics. HA is a hydrophilic compound that attracts water, and as a result, binds water continuously while it is metabolized, maintaining volume until its degradation.[21]

The lower orbital rim and the tear trough are common sites for filler use. A prominent tear trough deformity is characterized by a sunken appearance of the globe that results in a dark shadow over the lower eyelid, creating "under-eye circles."[22] The key is to inject small volumes; overcorrection should be avoided (**Fig. 5**). When treating midface volume loss, it should be performed first, because this may reduce the tear trough appearance and the amount of filler needed for the tear trough.

Volume augmentation of the upper eyelid can be accomplished by using HA or autologous fat transplant. It is usually injected in the postseptal area with slightly more volume placed in the lateral portion to provide more fullness.[1] The brow can be filled at a deeper level leading to elevation of the upper eyelid. Autologous fat transplant is biocompatible, naturally integrates into tissues without producing an inflammatory reaction, and potentially can be permanent

Overall, fillers can be a great adjunct to other procedures, such as BoNT injections, and with proper knowledge and experience can produce effective results.

DISCUSSION

There are a variety of treatment options that can be used for periorbital rejuvenation. Examining the severity of aging and patient expectations is important before selecting the best therapeutic option. Minimal photodamage with superficial rhytides can respond well to topical therapy and superficial chemical resurfacing. Moderate photodamage with deeper rhytides should be treated with medium depth peels or Er:YAG laser resurfacing. The use of the carbon dioxide laser as well as BoNT injections and fillers can be used to improve deep rhytides and severe photodamaged skin surface.

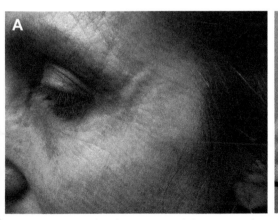
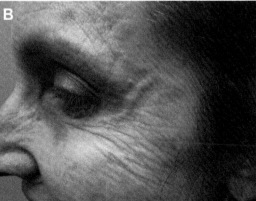

Fig. 4. (A) Two weeks after neuromodulator use to lateral canthal lines at repose. (B) With smiling, inferior rhytides accentuated by lateral cheek movement.

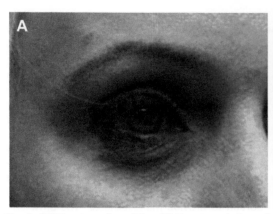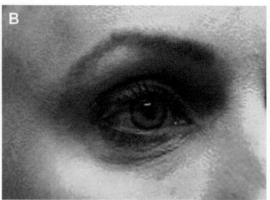

Fig. 5. (*A*) Tear trough prefiller. (*B*) Tear trough 3 weeks after injection with 0.5 mL HA filler.

REFERENCES

1. Glaser DA, Patel U. Enhancing the eyes: use of minimally invasive techniques for periorbital rejuvenation. J Drugs Dermatol 2010;9(8):s118–28.
2. Bucay VW, Day D. Adjunctive skin care of the brow and periorbital region. Clin Plast Surg 2013; 40:225–36.
3. Rubin MG. Chemical peels. Procedures in cosmetic dermatology. Amsterdam: Elsevier Inc; 2006. p. 1–12.
4. Jackson A. Chemical peels. Facial Plast Surg 2014; 30(1):26–34.
5. Hassan KM, Benedetto AV. Facial skin rejuvenation: ablative laser resurfacing, chemical peels, or photodynamic therapy? Facts and controversies. Clin Dermatol 2013;31(6):737–40.
6. Brodland DG, Cullimore KC, Roenigk RK, et al. Depths of chemexfoliation induced by various concentrations and application techniques of trichloroacetic acid in a porcine model. J Dermatol Surg Oncol 1989;15(9):967–71.
7. Nikalji N, Godse K, Sakhiya J, et al. Complications of medium depth and deep chemical peels. J Cutan Aesthet Surg 2012;5(4):254–60.
8. Brauer JA, Patel U, Hale EK. Laser skin resurfacing, chemical peels, and other cutaneous treatments of the brow and upper lid. Clin Plast Surg 2013;40(1): 91–9.
9. Shook BA, Hruza GJ. Periorbital ablative and nonablative resurfacing. Facial Plast Surg Clin North Am 2005;13(4):571–82.
10. Alster TS, Bellew SG. Improvement of dermatochalasis and periorbital rhytides with a high-energy pulsed CO2 laser: a retrospective study. Dermatol Surg 2004;30(4Pt 1):483–7.
11. Harboe B, Geronemus RG. Eyelid tightening by CO2 fractional laser, alternative to blepharoplasty. Dermatol Surg 2014;40(12):S137–41.
12. Fitzpatrick RE, Rostan EF, Marchell N. Collagen tightening induced by carbon dioxide laser versus erbium:YAG laser. Lasers Surg Med 2000;27(5): 395–403.
13. Bisson MA, Grover R, Grobbelaar AO. Long-term results of facial rejuvenation by carbon dioxide laser resurfacing using a quantitative method of assessment. Br J Plast Surg 2002;55:652–6.
14. Caniglia RJ. Erbium:YAG laser skin resurfacing. Facial Plast Surg Clin North Am 2004;12(3):373–7.
15. Alexiades-Armenakas MR, Dover JS, Arndt KA. The spectrum of laser skin resurfacing: nonablative, fractional, and ablative laser resurfacing. Dermatology 2008;58(5):719–37.
16. Fitzpatrick RE, Geronemus R, Goldberg D, et al. Multicenter study of noninvasive radiofrequency for periorbital tissue tightening. Lasers Surg Med 2003;33:232–42.
17. Carniol PJ, Hamilton MM, Carniol ET. Current status of fractional laser resurfacing. JAMA Facial Plast Surg 2015;17(5):360–6.
18. Erickson BP, Lee WW, Cohen J, et al. The role of neurotoxins in the periorbital and midfacial areas. Facial Plast Surg Clin North Am 2015;23(2):243–55.
19. Kane MAC. Nonsurgical periorbital and brow rejuvenation. Plast Reconstr Surg 2015;135(1):63–71.
20. Zimbler MS, Holds JB, Kokoska MS, et al. Effect of botulinum toxin pretreatment on laser resurfacing results: a prospective, randomized, blinded trial. Arch Facial Plast Surg 2001;3(3):165–9.
21. Lee S, Yen MT. Injectable hyaluronic acid fillers for periorbital rejuvenation. Int Ophthalmol Clin 2013; 53(3):1–9.
22. Sharad J. Dermal fillers for the treatment of tear trough deformity: a review of anatomy, treatment techniques, and their outcomes. J Cutan Aesthet Surg 2012;5(4):229–38.

Correction of Eyelid Crease Asymmetry and Ptosis

Steven M. Couch, MD, FACS

KEYWORDS

• Ptosis • Levator advancement • MMCR • Eyelid crease • Pretarsal platform

KEY POINTS

- Involutional changes with levator aponeurotic dehiscence is the most common cause of blepharoptosis, which presents with low margin-to-reflex distance, elevated eyelid crease, and normal levator function.
- Pretarsal platform is a complex anatomic structure defined by the anatomic eyelid crease and preseptal skin, fat, and brow positions.
- Precise surgical levator advancement can lead to appropriate marginal contour, symmetric height and allows exact eyelid crease management.
- Muller muscle conjunctiva resection is an effective, precise surgical procedure that requires no intraoperative patient interaction for improvement of ptosis and eyelid crease asymmetry.
- Eyelid crease creation and symmetry improvement can be achieved with or without ptosis repair and involves deep fixation of pretarsal anterior lamellae to the levator aponeurosis.

INTRODUCTION

The complex anatomy of the upper eyelid is not only responsible for the upper eyelid position superior to the visual axis, but also contributes to the aesthetically pleasing lines of the eyelid margin and eyelid crease, and their relationship to the brow. The function of the upper eyelid is ocular protection and tear dispersion over the eye. Upper eyelid retractors, which are responsible for upper eyelid height and excursion, include the levator muscle and its aponeurosis, Muller muscle, and limited functions from the frontalis muscle (**Fig. 1**). The levator muscle, which is primarily responsible for upper eyelid height and excursion, is innervated by the oculomotor nerve after its origination on the sphenoid bone in the posterior orbit. The skeletal muscle of the levator palpebrae superioris transitions into an aponeurosis after passing through the Whitnall check ligament in the superior orbit. Traditionally, the upper eyelid crease is thought to derive from the insertion of the levator aponeurosis fibers into the anterior lamellae of the eyelid. Muller muscle is an involuntary, sympathetically innervated, smooth muscle, which originates on the undersurface of the levator muscle and inserts at the superior edge of tarsus. The peripheral arcade of eyelid is an excellent landmark as it sits just above the tarsus, sandwiched between the levator aponeurosis and Muller muscle. The orbicularis muscle is a sphincter within the anterior lamellae and is responsible for eyelid protraction.

The ideal upper eyelid exhibits a gentle curve with acute medial angle, peaks as it extends laterally beyond the pupil, and gently tapers as it extends temporally.[1–3] Centrally, the upper eyelid margin commonly falls just below the superior

Disclosure Statement: The author has nothing to disclose.
Department of Ophthalmology and Visual Sciences, Washington University in St. Louis, 660 South Euclid Avenue, Campus Box 8096, St Louis, MO 63110, USA
E-mail address: CouchS@vision.wustl.edu

Facial Plast Surg Clin N Am 24 (2016) 153–162
http://dx.doi.org/10.1016/j.fsc.2015.12.009
1064-7406/16/$ – see front matter © 2016 Elsevier Inc. All rights reserved.

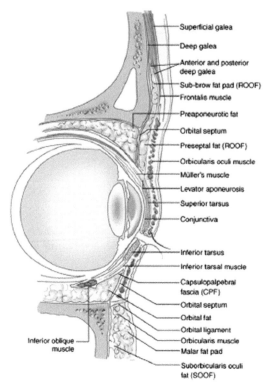

Fig. 1. Cross-sectional anatomy of the upper and lower eyelid. Upper eyelid retractors, including the levator aponeurosis and Muller muscle, are visible. Note insertion of the orbital septum onto the levator aponeurosis and the importance of the preaponeurotic fat in the identification of the levator aponeurosis. (*From* Most SP, Mobley SR, Larrabee WF Jr. Anatomy of the eyelids [review]. Facial Plast Surg Clin North Am 2005;13:486–92; with permission.)

limbus but still well above the central visual axis. The healthy upper eyelid is full without significant fat protrusion.[4,5] The complex relationship of the upper eyelid not only involves the height of the margin in relation to the visual axis, but also the stature of the pretarsal platform. Classically in most anatomic textbooks, the insertion of fibers from the levator aponeurosis into the orbicularis muscle and skin are responsible for the formation and maintenance of the eyelid crease. Functionally, the upper eyelid crease is formed at the "buckle point" of the upper eyelid skin where the nonfixated preseptal and orbital skin meets the well-fixated pretarsal anterior lamellae.[6] Because of differences in the amount of excess eyelid skin and fat, in addition to brow architecture, the anatomic upper eyelid crease does not always correspond with the height of the pretarsal platform. Eyelid creases and secondarily the pretarsal platform can take on multiple shapes, including tapered, semilunar, and parallel.

Compensatory brow elevation is commonly noted in patients with acquired blepharoptosis and can be noted not only as brow asymmetry but also frontalis muscle stimulation on the elevated side. Frequently, the brow will achieve normal height following repair of blepharoptosis. Symmetry is the key to the cosmetically appealing upper eyelid. Not only is the upper eyelid height evenness crucial, but the shape, pretarsal platform height, eyelid crease curvature, and brow position are all equally important in aesthetic eyelid evaluation.[7,8]

Blepharoptosis of the upper eyelid is diagnosed when the upper eyelid margin to corneal light reflex distance (MRD) is abnormally low and can occur in one eye or both eyes.[9,10] Ptosis is commonly secondary to senile involution, but in some cases can have secondary myogenic, neurogenic, or mechanical causes. Dehiscence of the levator aponeurosis causing ptosis can occur as an age-related involutional change, but is more prevalent in contact lens wearers and patients who have undergone ocular surgery. Measurement of eyelid elevator function remains one of the best differentiating factors for ptosis etiologies. Unlike other etiologies, levator function is normal in patients with involutional ptosis despite levator aponeurotic disinsertion.

Eyelid crease asymmetry is commonly associated with blepharoptosis but can have other congenital, anatomic, or ethnic etiologies.[10] Commonly with levator dehiscence, the pretarsal platform will expand secondary to elevation of the eyelid crease (**Fig. 2**). Despite normal MRD, congenital and anatomic eyelid crease asymmetries are common and may require surgical correction. Aesthetically, symmetry of eyelid MRD and contour are important; however, height of pretarsal platform may be more important for some patients.[11,12]

PREOPERATIVE PLANNING AND PREPARATION

Ptosis repair can be desired for several different reasons, including visual obstruction, heavy

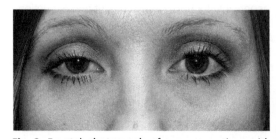

Fig. 2. Frontal photograph of a young patient with involutional ptosis of the right upper eyelid. Note elevation of right upper eyelid crease, compensatory brow elevation, and diminished MRD.

sensation, contact lens fitting, and cosmetic improvement. Ideal results of surgery depend on appropriate surgical candidate selection, preoperative planning, and surgical technique. Consideration of patient concerns, etiology of complaints, anatomic findings, systemic or ocular comorbidities, and goals of surgery should be intertwined to develop a surgical plan. A clear understanding of patients' concerns will allow the surgeon to evaluate the likelihood of achieving the desired goals. Patients may complain of visual obstruction, eyelid heaviness, or even droopy eyelid, which may relate to a low MRD, excessive eyelid skin, or even pretarsal platform asymmetry. A mutual understanding should be achieved between the patient and surgeon with a clear expectation of anticipated surgical outcomes. If possible, poor surgical candidates, those with unrealistic expectations, and patients with worrisome secondary diagnoses inducing ptosis should be avoided.

One goal of evaluating patients with upper eyelid ptosis is to exclude secondary worrisome causes that may affect patient health or surgical candidacy. Besides an in-depth evaluation of the patient's complaints and systemic assessment, several ophthalmic findings should be appraised, including MRD, levator excursion, skin crease, eyelid height variability, orbicularis strength, and Bell phenomenon.[13] The MRD is best measured in primary gaze with a millimeter ruler and a dim flashlight. Fixation of the patient's gaze onto the light allows the most accurate assessment. Levator excursion is the most clinically useful assessment as to the health of the levator, and the measurement is taken for the amount of movement of the eyelid margin from extreme downgaze to extreme upgaze. Isolation of the eyelid with

brow immobilization and avoiding head movement will provide the best assessment. Normal excursion ranges from 12 to 18 mm. Suspicion of a secondary cause for ptosis should be considered if levator movement is less than 12 mm or significantly different between eyes (**Fig. 3**).

Anatomic and visible eyelid crease should be measured in addition to amount of excess skin and fat. Typical eyelid creases in Occidental adults range from 6 to 8 mm in men and 8 to 10 mm in women. Elevated upper eyelid creases are commonly seen with ptosis caused by aponeurotic dehiscence. Absent, excessively low or multiplication of the eyelid crease can be seen in Asian patients. Brow position is important to note before surgical intervention in the eyelids. Significant variability in the eyelid height, either historically or during the examination, may signify an underlying medical cause including myasthenia gravis. Patients with poor orbicularis strength, lagophthalmos, limited ocular motility, or severe dry eyes are likely not optimal ptosis repair or upper eyelid surgery candidates. A thorough ophthalmic evaluation is needed before considering upper eyelid ptosis repair. Assessments of tear film, corneal dryness, previous surgeries (including refractive surgery), and other ophthalmic pathology are necessary to avoid complications. Patients with normal levator function, normal or elevated eyelid crease, good Bell phenomenon, good orbicularis function, normal ocular alignment, and healthy tear films are typically good candidates for surgery.

Instillation of phenylephrine (2.5% or 10.0%) into the eye, twice over 5 minutes, is paramount for patients who you would consider for Muller muscle conjunctival resection (MMCR) (**Fig. 4**). Phenylephrine stimulates the sympathetically stimulated

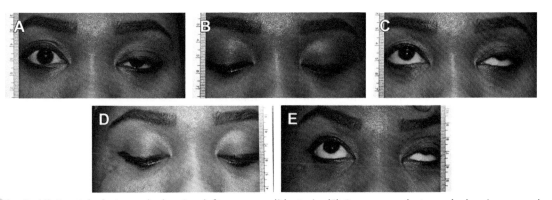

Fig. 3. (A) Frontal photograph showing left upper eyelid ptosis. (B) Downgaze photograph showing normal downgaze excursion on the right. (C) Normal upgaze levator function of more than 15 mm. (D) Slight left upper eyelid retraction on downgaze, suggestive of diminished levator function. (E) Diminished levator function noted on upgaze. Note brow fixation to allow isolation of levator excursion. Diminished levator function is suggestive of a secondary cause for ptosis.

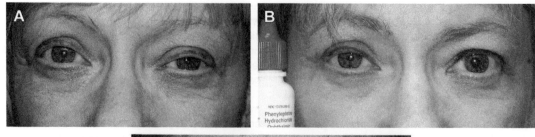

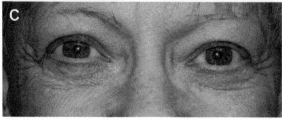

Fig. 4. (*A*) Left upper eyelid involutional ptosis. (*B*) After instillation of 2.5% phenylephrine into the left eye, the patient notices significant elevation in the left upper eyelid, slightly above the desired result. (*C*) Following successful left upper eyelid MMCR.

Muller muscle to contract and therefore causes elevation of the eyelid margin. Following phenylephrine administration, the MRD is reassessed and if noted to be raised to a normal level or above, they may be good candidates for MMCR. The degree of ptosis and level of response can allow the surgeon to algorithmically plan the amount of resection during the surgery (**Table 1**). Patients

who do not elevate or do not elevate enough following phenylephrine instillation would likely be better candidates for levator advancement.

The Herring law explains that extraocular muscles, including the levator muscle, are innervated with equal intensity by the brain. In some patients with ptosis, elevation of the upper eyelid either in unilateral ptosis or those with asymmetric ptosis will induce ptosis on the contralateral side.[14] Preoperatively this can be occasionally predicted during manual or phenylephrine-induced elevation of the ptotic eyelid (**Fig. 5**). If the contralateral eyelid significantly drops during preoperative evaluation, the patient should be advised of its possibility postoperatively and either an adjustment should be made intraoperatively or bilateral surgery should be considered. In one study, this was shown to occur in up to 10% of patients evaluated and treated for ptosis.[14]

PTOSIS REPAIR

Unlike standard upper eyelid blepharoplasty, which has a limited effect on the dynamic eyelid function, ptosis repair is commonly considered a "deeper" surgery, which has profound effects on function and therefore appearance. Typically, ptosis repair is more time consuming, complex, and depends on a greater detailed surgical plan than blepharoplasty. Surgical intervention for blepharoptosis depends on patient preference and surgeon training and preference, along with goals of surgery. Surgery is commonly performed in an operating suite and can be accomplished with a range of anesthesia choices including strictly local

Table 1
Summary of each major study evaluating algorithms for the amount of resection to perform during a Muller muscle conjunctival resection based on eyelid response preoperatively to phenylephrine

Article	Proposed Algorithm
Putterman and Urist,[18] 1975	8.25 mm of resection, +1 mm for undercorrection and −1 for overcorrection with phenylephrine
Weinstein & Buerger,[20] 1982	4 mm for 1-mm ptosis, 6 mm for 1.5-mm, 10 mm for 2-mm, 12 mm for <3-mm ptosis
Dresner,[19] 2001	8-mm resection for 2-mm ptosis, vary resection by 1 mm for each 0.25 mm away from 2 mm of ptosis
Perry et al,[21] 2002	9 mm of resection for everyone + tarsal resection at 1:1-mm ratio for each mm of undercorrection following phenylephrine instillation

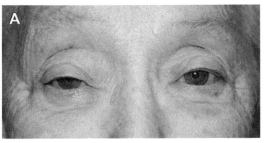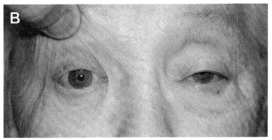

Fig. 5. (*A*) Bilateral upper eyelid ptosis with profound functional complaints on the right. (*B*) Manual elevation of the right upper eyelid induces further left upper eyelid ptosis through the Herring response. This may be an indication of the need for bilateral surgery in a patient with unilateral complaints.

anesthesia and general anesthesia. With levator-advancement surgery, patient cooperation during surgery is a key to success, thus light sedation is preferred, whereas posterior approach ptosis repair can be performed under any range of sedation, including general anesthesia.

Severity of ptosis and degree of levator excursion also should be considered when deciding technique for ptosis repair. Patients with mild, moderate, and severe ptosis can be managed with levator advancement, whereas those with moderate to severe ptosis may be best avoided with MMCR. Levator advancement surgery can be performed on patients with moderate to good levator function, but MMCR should be reserved only for patients with good levator function.

EXTERNAL PTOSIS REPAIR

External levator advancement is one of the most commonly performed oculoplastic procedures and is traditionally considered the procedure of choice, as it addresses the underlying cause of involutional ptosis.[15–17] Typically performed under local anesthesia with light sedation, patient participation is key for success in external levator advancement surgery. Excessive drowsiness, poor patient participation, or general anesthesia typically will lead to an abnormality in the patient's eyelid height or contour and therefore symmetry. Preoperatively, the patient's eyelid height and contour are evaluated in the sitting and supine laying positions. Eyelid incisions are marked, which can be performed through small incisions (<10 mm), large incisions over the entire eyelid length, or can be combined with a blepharoplasty (**Fig. 6**). Typically the incision line should correspond with the level of the anticipated eyelid crease. Light sedation can be administered early in the case as local anesthesia is infiltrated into the upper eyelid. Care should be taken to inject identical amounts and locations in bilateral cases and avoid an injection-induced hematoma. Drapes

are applied with care taken to avoid traction on the eyebrows or upper eyelid skin.

Skin incision is made, and if a blepharoplasty is to be performed, skin excision is performed before the ptosis repair. A plane is commonly elevated between the orbicularis muscle and the orbital septum 5 mm above the eyelid crease. The orbital septum is then incised and widely opened with careful attention to the underlying levator aponeurosis. Preaponeurotic fat is then dissected free of the levator aponeurosis and can be cauterized for retraction or resected as desired. If the levator aponeurosis is dehisced, thin tissue is seen with a white condensation within the aponeurosis superior to the tarsal edge. An incision is made in the levator aponeurosis just behind the cut edge of the pretarsal orbicularis to expose the anterior aspect of the tarsal plate. The anterior face of the tarsus is exposed, typically just wide enough to allow suture placement. Careful dissection is performed under the levator aponeurosis to separate it from the Muller muscle with cautious avoidance of the peripheral arcade. A nonabsorbable suture is passed partial thickness through the anterior aspect of the tarsus and then in a horizontal mattress fashion used to advance the levator aponeurosis cut edge. Precise suture placement within the tarsus in the horizontal and vertical dimension along with length of suture pass will determine contour of the upper eyelid. Traditionally, the suture pass should be several millimeters wide and placed within a few millimeters of the superior tarsal edge just medial to the proposed highest point of margin elevation. Although in many cases, single suture advancement can be performed and an appropriate height and contour achieved. The suture is secured with a temporary knot. If bilateral surgery is being performed, the identical exposure is executed on the contralateral side. Eyelid height and contour are evaluated in both sitting and supine positions. In addition to evaluating height in primary gaze, symmetry can be also appreciated and adjustments made following evaluation in

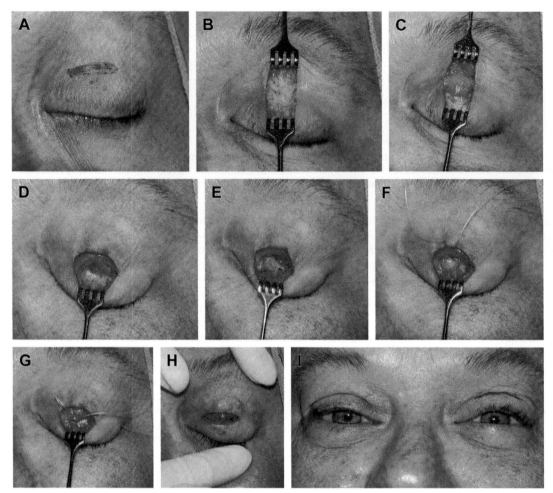

Fig. 6. (*A*) Incision made at level of anticipated crease. (*B*) Orbicularis muscle incised and dissection performed between the orbicularis and orbital septum. (*C*) Orbital septum is widely opened and silky preaponeurotic fat exposed. (*D*) Incision made in attenuated levator aponeurosis to expose the anterior tarsal plate. (*E*) Partial-thickness suture (5–0 double-armed Mersiline) placed in the tarsal plate just medial to the pupil. (*F*) Horizontal mattress advancement of the levator aponeurosis. (*G*) Temporary knot secured to assess eyelid height and contour. (*H*) Crease fixation and levator secured to the pretarsal orbicularis muscle. (*I*) Intraoperative evaluation of left upper eyelid showing good contour and slight overcorrection.

upgaze and downgaze. Contour irregularities may be best assessed with vertical gaze. Excess stimulation of Muller muscle secondary to local anesthesia with epinephrine or manipulation may lead to intraoperative height or contour abnormalities that can be counteracted by stretch on the eyelid and temporarily secured sutures during the height evaluation.

Suture adjustment, placement of additional sutures, or further dissection is performed as needed to achieve identical height and contour. Once sutures have achieved satisfactory levels, they are permanently secured. In general, patients undergoing unilateral surgery should have eyelid margins placed up to 1 mm higher than their contralateral eyelid height, and patients undergoing bilateral surgery should be equal with eyelid heights no higher than 1 mm lower the superior limbus.

Excess advanced levator aponeurosis is excised. Eyelid crease formation is performed with small-caliber absorbable sutures securing the cut edge of the pretarsal orbicularis muscle to the cut, advanced edge of the levator aponeurosis. Microscopic marginal contour or eyelid crease abnormalities can be corrected with precise crease-forming suture. Skin closure is then performed (**Fig. 7**).

INTERNAL PTOSIS REPAIR

MMCR is a popular ptosis repair technique that was first described by Putterman and Urist[18] in

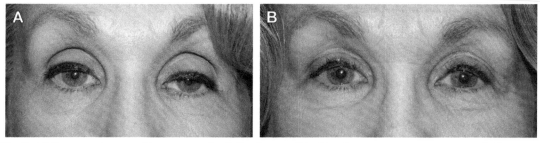

Fig. 7. (*A*) Preoperative and (*B*) postoperative following small incision levator advancement; note rigid contact lenses are highly associated with progressive involutional ptosis.

1975 as a modification of the Fasanella-Servat procedure. MMCR requires no intraoperative patient cooperation and can provide an excellent ptosis repair in patients with mild to moderate ptosis and good levator function. Preoperative assessment following phenylephrine instillation is key to the decisions made for surgical repair. Multiple nomograms for amount of posterior resection to be performed have been created and rely on amount of ptosis preoperatively and quantification of the response to phenylephrine (see **Table 1**).[19–21]

MMCR can be performed under local or general anesthesia and can be performed simultaneously with an external upper eyelid blepharoplasty. The frontal nerve block is administered using injectable local anesthesia with epinephrine. In addition, a small amount of anesthesia is administered into the pretarsal skin. Occasionally, a superior fornix injection may be required for adequate anesthesia. A traction suture is commonly placed in the tarsal edge and the upper eyelid is everted over a Desmarres retractor (**Fig. 8**). The conjunctival side is evaluated, and then, using the preoperatively decided nomogram, the amount of conjunctiva to be resected is measured starting just above the superior edge of the tarsus. Either a marking pen is used to define the entire area of resection or a traction suture is placed half the distance of resection to aid in clamp placement. A toothed forceps

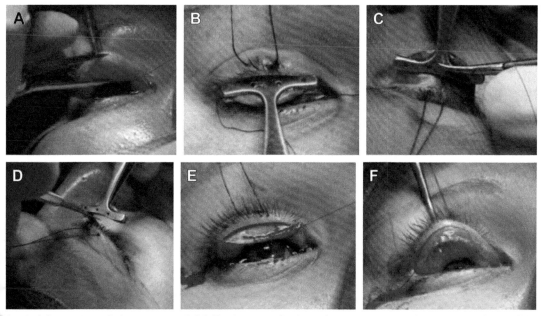

Fig. 8. (*A*) Eversion of the upper eyelid following anesthesia and traction suture placement, marking of the amount of conjunctiva to be excised. (*B*) Placement of the MMCR clamp with care taken to avoid levator aponeurosis and skin incorporation. (*C*) Running of suture from temporally to medially just below the clamp. (*D*) Excision of clamped tissue with #15 Bard Parker blade passed between suture and clamp with blade angled toward clamp. (*E*) Resection bed following tissue removal. (*F*) Suture is then passed in a running fashion through the cut edges temporally, externalized, and tied. (*Courtesy of* Morris Hartstein, MD, Raanana, Israel.)

is then used to separate the Muller muscle/conjunctiva complex from the underlying levator aponeurosis. A Putterman Mullerectomy clamp is used to secure the marked tissue with care taken to avoid capturing the levator within the clamped material. As the blades of the clamp engage the tissue, the Desmarres retractor is rotated out from the eyelid. The skin is distracted from the clamp to ensure no skin or levator aponeurosis is incorporated in the demarcated tissue. The clamp is then locked with the secured conjunctiva and Muller muscle only incorporated within the clamp. A double-armed 5 to 0 plain gut or 6 to 0 chromic gut suture is then passed in a horizontal mattress fashion just below the clamp from the temporal aspect of the eyelid nasally. The suture is then tightened to ensure no loops are present, and a blade is passed with the bevel pointing toward the clamp just superior to the suture, along the undersurface of the clamp, transecting the clamped tissues. The nasal arm of suture is then run temporally in a continuous fashion through the cut edges with incorporation of the tarsal edge, externalized through the eyelid and secured externally.

SURGICAL CREASE FORMATION

The anatomic crease of the upper eyelid occurs at the junction point of the fixated pretarsal anterior lamellae and the nonfixated upper eyelid/brow skin. The visible pretarsal platform not only relies on the position of the anatomic crease, but also the bulk in the upper eyelid and brow. Symmetry is achieved when the visible platform matches between the 2 eyelids, but it requires identical amounts of upper eyelid and brow tissue. Traditionally, well-defined creases have a feminizing characterization and many surgeons have used deep crease fixation in women or Asian upper eyelid surgery.

As upper eyelid ptosis is improved by either levator advancement or MMCR, the typical by-product is depression of the eyelid crease and subsequent shortening of the tarsal platform. Incision planning and crease fixation will determine crease height following external ptosis repair or blepharoplasty. In his American Ophthalmologic Society thesis, Goldberg and Lew[6] described cosmetic outcomes of MMCR surgery. They showed a significant decrease in the tarsal platform show, unless concurrent blepharoplasty was performed, then the tarsal platform was elevated.

The goal of anatomic crease fixation involves the fixation of the mobile pretarsal anterior lamellae, which traditionally involves its attachment to the levator aponeurosis before skin closure. A "soft" crease fixation can be achieved if the levator aponeurosis is captured during running or interrupted skin-closing sutures. Rigid crease fixation may require layered closure of the eyelid with deeper sutures firmly adhering the anterior lamellae to the levator (**Fig. 9**). After blepharoplasty or ptosis repairs, a 7 to 0 Vicryl suture can be placed in the cut edge of the pretarsal orbicularis and attached to the levator aponeurosis before skin closure. Occasionally, redundant preaponeurotic fascia can be excised, providing a clean plane for deep suturing of the pretarsal orbicularis to the levator aponeurosis. Depending on the extent of crease fixation desired, a few sutures can be used in the central eyelid or multiple sutures may be necessary across the entire length of the eyelid (**Fig. 10**). Precise surgical treatment of Asian blepharoplasty is outside of the scope of this article, but it requires deep, defined crease fixation across the entire eyelid.

Postoperative Care

Following upper eyelid ptosis repair, ice and head elevation are important, along with application of topical antibiotic ointment to incisions. Patients

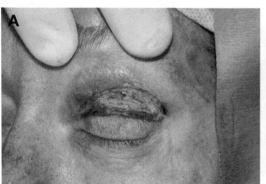
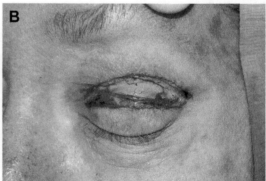

Fig. 9. (*A*) Intraoperative left upper eyelid during blepharoplasty with loose anterior lamellae. (*B*) Intraoperative tightening of the pretarsal orbicularis muscle to the levator aponeurosis with rigid fixation of the anterior lamellae and therefore crease.

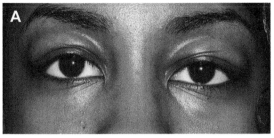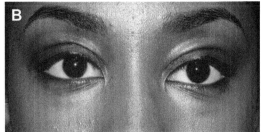

Fig. 10. (*A*) Young woman with known blepharochalasis syndrome with loose anterior lamellae. (*B*) Postoperative following minimal skin resection but rigid crease fixation and lacrimal gland repositioning.

are instructed to call if they experience severe pain, excessive bleeding, or vision concerns. At the first postoperative visit, eyelid height, contour, closure, and corneal status are evaluated. Complications following MMCR could include pyogenic granulomas or corneal abrasions. Cutaneous sutures are removed and patients are reevaluated several months after repair.

Excessive abnormalities may require revision, including early postoperative levator aponeurosis adjustment in patients with significant eyelid malposition. Early postoperative adjustment can be performed within several weeks following aponeurotic advancement and may involve opening of the incision and suture adjustment or replacement. Early postoperative adjustment following MMCR is difficult and rare. Final eyelid height following MMCR may not be achieved for several months after surgery and if not desirable may be amenable to either repeat MMCR or levator advancement.

SUMMARY

External anatomy of the upper eyelid involves not only the margin height in reference to the globe, but also the marginal contour, eyelid crease stature, and the tarsal platform show. When patients complain of droopy eyelids, they may be referring to excess eyelid skin, margin height, or even differences in the amount of tarsal platform show. During the evaluation of patients with ptosis, it is important to specifically assess levator function, ocular motility, and Bell phenomenon, and in many cases, the Herring phenomenon can be elucidated before surgery. In some patients, levator advancement may provide the best option for functional and cosmetic outcomes, especially in those concurrently undergoing blepharoplasty or those who require correction of moderate to severe ptosis. Although technically easier, the MMCR is highly dependent on algorithms for amount of conjunctiva and Muller muscle resection, many of which have been published with wide variability.

Because the levator aponeurosis is partially responsible for the eyelid crease height, correction of ptosis will commonly lead to improvement and address symmetry of the eyelid crease. In some patients, eyelid height is normal and pretarsal show is asymmetric and must be addressed with careful and deep crease fixation. A methodical assessment and precise surgical intervention for eyelid ptosis and crease asymmetries can lead to happy patients with excellent outcomes.

REFERENCES

1. Reilly MJ, Tomsic JA, Fernandez SJ, et al. Effect of facial rejuvenation surgery on perceived attractiveness, femininity, and personality. JAMA Facial Plast Surg 2015;17(3):202–7.
2. Ing E, Safarpour A, Ing T, et al. Ocular adnexal asymmetry in models: a magazine photograph analysis. Can J Ophthalmol 2006;41(2):175–82.
3. Tower RN, Soparkar CN, Patrinely JR. Perspectives on periocular asymmetry. Semin Plast Surg 2007; 21(1):18–23.
4. Massry GG. Ptosis repair for the cosmetic surgeon. Facial Plast Surg Clin North Am 2005; 13(4):533–9, vi.
5. Volpe CR, Ramirez OM. The beautiful eye. Facial Plast Surg Clin North Am 2005;13(4):493–504.
6. Goldberg RA, Lew H. Cosmetic outcome of posterior approach ptosis surgery (an American Ophthalmological Society thesis). Trans Am Ophthalmol Soc 2011;109:157–67.
7. Macdonald KI, Mendez AI, Hart RD, et al. Eyelid and brow asymmetry in patients evaluated for upper lid blepharoplasty. J Otolaryngol Head Neck Surg 2014;43(1):36.
8. Ellenbogen R, Swara N. Correction of asymmetrical upper eyelids by measured levator adhesion technique. Plast Reconstr Surg 1982;69(3):433–44.
9. Putterman AM. Margin reflex distance (MRD) 1, 2, and 3. Ophthal Plast Reconstr Surg 2012;28(4):308–11.
10. Murchison AP, Sires BA, Jian-Amadi A. Margin reflex distance in different ethnic groups. Arch Facial Plast Surg 2009;11(5):303–5.

11. Buchanan AG, Holds JB. The beautiful eye: perception of beauty in the periocular area. Chapter 3. In: Paul MD, Hovsepian RV, Rotunda AM, editors. Master techniques in blepharoplasty and periorbital rejuvenation. New York: Springer Science 1 Business Media; 2011. p. 25–9.

12. Patrocinio TG, Loredo BA, Arevalo CE, et al. Complications in blepharoplasty: how to avoid and manage them. Braz J Otorhinolaryngol 2011;77(3):322–7.

13. Small RG, Sabates NR, Burrows D. The measurement and definition of ptosis. Ophthal Plast Reconstr Surg 1989;5(3):171–5.

14. Bodian M. Lid droop following contralateral ptosis repair. Arch Ophthalmol 1982;100:1122–4.

15. Jones LT, Quickert MH, Wobig JL. The cure of ptosis by aponeurotic repair. Arch Ophthalmol 1978;93: 629–34.

16. Anderson RL. Aponeurotic ptosis repair. Arch Ophthalmol 1979;97:1123–8.

17. Older JJ. Levator aponeurotic surgery for the correction of acquired ptosis. Ophthalmology 1983;90:1056–9.

18. Putterman AM, Urist MJ. Müllers muscle conjunctival resection. Arch Ophthalmol 1975;93:619–23.

19. Dresner SC. Further modifications of Müller's muscle conjunctival resection procedure for blepharoptosis. Ophthal Plast Reconstr Surg 1991;7:114–22.

20. Weinstein GS, Buerger GF. The modification of Müller's muscle conjunctival resection operation for blepharoptosis. Am J Ophthalmol 1993;5:647–51.

21. Perry JD, Kadakia A, Foster JA. A new algorithm for ptosis repair using conjunctival mullerectomy with or without tarsectomy. Ophthal Plast Reconstr Surg 2002;18(6):426–9.

Lower Lid Malposition
Causes and Correction

Samuel Hahn, MD[a], Shaun C. Desai, MD[b],*

KEYWORDS

• Lower lid malposition • Lower lid retraction • Ectropion • Entropion • Horizontal lid laxity

KEY POINTS

- Correction of lower lid malposition requires intricate understanding of the trilamellar eyelid and lower lid–midface unit for selection of appropriate surgical techniques.
- Preoperative assessment of lower lid tone and position is critical, and horizontal lid tightening procedures should be considered if any preoperative lower lid laxity if noted.
- Transcutaneous approach for lower lid blepharoplasty has a higher risk of postblepharoplasty lower lid malposition than the transconjunctival approach, thus judicious skin/muscle excision is essential.
- Ectropion and entropion are multifactorial conditions that require careful understanding of cause to choose the appropriate surgical or nonsurgical treatment.

INTRODUCTION

Malposition of the lower eyelid is a challenging condition that can result from a host of causes. The consequence of lower lid malformation can widely range from aesthetically unpleasing but functionally harmless to devastating vision loss due to ocular complications. Understanding the causes of lower lid malposition will help determine the surgical or nonsurgical approaches required to best treat the malposition. Complete knowledge of the lower eyelid anatomy and appreciation of the lower eyelid–midface unit is important in determining the physiologic factors that contribute to lower eyelid malposition. The surgical techniques aimed at treating lower lid malposition require understanding the relationship of the trilamellar lower lid and the resultant deficiencies or constraints that result in lower lid malpositioning. Additional risk factors, such as horizontal laxity of the lid, that predispose lower lid malposition must be taken into account whenever lower eyelid surgery is considered. Failure to do so can result in postoperative lower lid retraction or ectropion that may be difficult to correct.

APPLIED ANATOMY OF THE LOWER EYELID

An intricate understanding of the complex lower lid anatomy is paramount for the treatment of lower lid malposition in eyelid surgery. The lower eyelid can be viewed as a dynamic structure suspended by a fibroligamentous sling that is supported by the medial and lateral canthal tendons, the tarsus, lower lid retractors, and orbicularis oculi muscle (**Fig. 1**). The margin of the lower eyelid sits at or just above the level of the inferior limbus, and the tarsus approximates the globe. The lateral canthal tendon sits roughly 2 to 4 mm superior to the medial canthal tendon, forming a lateral canthal angle of roughly 60°.[1]

From anterior to posterior, the lower eyelid can be divided into the anterior, middle, and posterior lamellae. The anterior lamella consists of the thinnest skin in the body with no underlying subcutaneous fat opposing the orbicularis oculi

[a] Facial Plastic and Reconstructive Surgery, Department of Otolaryngology, Head and Neck Surgery, Washington University School of Medicine, 1020 North Mason Road, Suite 205, Creve Coeur, MO 63141, USA; [b] Division of Facial Plastic and Reconstructive Surgery, Department of Otolaryngology, Head and Neck Surgery, Johns Hopkins University School of Medicine, 6420 Rockledge Drive, Suite 4920, Bethesda, MD 20817, USA
* Corresponding author.
E-mail address: sdesai27@jhmi.edu

Facial Plast Surg Clin N Am 24 (2016) 163–171
http://dx.doi.org/10.1016/j.fsc.2015.12.006
1064-7406/16/$ – see front matter © 2016 Elsevier Inc. All rights reserved.

facialplastic.theclinics.com

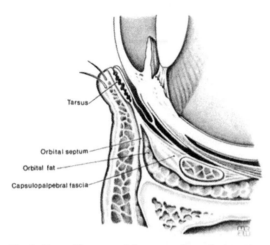

Tarsus

Orbital septum

Orbital fat

Capsulopalpebral fascia

Fig. 1. Normal lower eyelid anatomy. Note the insertion of the orbital septum on the capsulopalpebral fascia. (*From* Patipa M. The evaluation and management of lower eyelid retraction following cosmetic surgery. Plast Reconstr Surg 2000;106(2):439; with permission.)

muscle. The orbicularis muscle can be further divided into the palpebral and orbital orbicularis muscle. The palpebral orbicularis muscle plays an important role in lower lid apposition to the globe and lacrimal pumping. The middle lamella refers to the orbital septum acting as a supportive layer dividing the anterior and posterior lamellae.[2] The posterior lamella is composed of the tarsus superiorly and the lower lid retractor, otherwise known as the capsulopalpebral fascia, inferiorly as well as the palpebral conjunctiva. The interaction between the distinct layers of the lower eyelid contributes to the overall contour and position of the lower eyelid. Understanding this trilamellar model of the lower eyelid will help surgeons recognize the numerous factors that can affect the positioning of the lower eyelid.

Understanding the anatomic relationship of the lower eyelid–midface unit is important in recognizing the role midface descent can play in lower lid malpositioning. The suborbicularis oculi fat lies inferior to the orbital rim and is contiguous with the malar fat pad. The malar fat pad is a triangular structure with the apex positioned over the malar eminence.[3] As the midface ages, there is bony remodeling, descent of the malar fat pad secondary to gravity, as well as fat atrophy, which result in lower eyelid descent and malposition due to loss of support.

PREOPERATIVE ASSESSMENT FOR LOWER EYELID SURGERY

Careful and thorough preoperative assessment is crucial for proper operative planning before any

lower eyelid procedure. Preoperative evaluation should start with a thorough medical history to evaluate for risk factors for lower eyelid malposition. Medical history should include history of any ocular conditions, thyroid disease, and prior facial trauma. A detailed surgical history should also be obtained focusing on prior orbital or midface surgery and facial rejuvenation procedures. Symptoms of dry eyes, epiphora, or ocular irritation should also be noted in the examination.

Examination of the lower eyelid should start with assessment of the lower lid position in relation to the globe by measuring the relative positions of the lateral and medial canthus and the margin-reflex distance 2. Patients should be asked to close their eyelids and raise their eyebrows to observe for any lagophthalmos. If present, ocular examination may reveal conjunctival irritation or keratitis. Forced eyelid closure can assess for orbicularis strength and facial nerve function.

Assessment of Horizontal Lid Laxity

Assessment of the degree of horizontal laxity and tone of the lower eyelid can be performed through the lid distraction and snap test. The lid distraction test is performed by gently grasping and pulling the lower lid away from the globe; distraction greater than 8 mm is suggestive of excessive laxity. The snap test or lid retraction test is performed by retracting the lower eyelid inferiorly and assessing the speed and position of the recoil of the lid when released. The lower eyelid should spring back to its natural position without blinking. A slow or incomplete return to the original lid position indicates decreased tone of the orbicularis muscle and excessive laxity of the tarsoligamentous sling. Patients exhibiting signs concerning for lower lid laxity will need to have horizontal lid tightening to prevent postoperative lower lid malposition and subsequent ocular complications. In addition to assessment of lower lid laxity, evaluation of the lower lid mobility will guide the surgeon to contributing factors to lower lid malposition. Manual elevation of the lower eyelid can assess for any inferior tethering or shortening of the lower eyelid, which may require release and spacer grafting for correction.

Assessment of Globe Position

An evaluation of the globe position in relation to the inferior orbital rim on a profile view is important to assess the risk for postoperative lower lid malposition. A patient with a negative vector configuration, a globe positioned anterior to the orbital rim, is likely to have less midfacial support and is at higher risk for lower lid malpositioning after lower lid blepharoplasty. In patients with concern for exophthalmos, a Hertel exophthalmometer can be used to measure the distance from the lateral orbital rim to the anterior globe. Patients with measurements greater than 17 mm are at higher risk for postoperative lid malposition with fat excision or lid-tightening procedures and may require additional orbicularis suspension or spacer graft to prevent malposition.[4,5]

Assessment of the Midface

The lower eyelid is intimately associated with the midface, and descent of the midface can result in magnified lower lid malpositioning. Assessment of the midface should be performed preoperatively by assessing the lower lid and malar contour following finger repositioning of the lower eyelid. Persistent central lower eyelid retraction or tension in conjunction with malar flattening is suggestive of midface descent that may require repositioning of the cheek fat pad or malar implants to fully correct the lower lid malpositioning.[6] Recognizing preexisting risk factors for postoperative lower eyelid malposition in patients undergoing lower eyelid surgery is essential for preventing postoperative complications.

LOWER LID MALPOSITION: PATHOPHYSIOLOGY AND TREATMENT

Lower lid malposition encompasses a continuum of lower eyelid conditions that range from lower lid retraction to ectropion and entropion. The causes of lower lid malpositioning are many, and understanding the pathophysiology and anatomic abnormalities that contribute to lower lid malpositioning is essential to planning a successful intervention.

LOWER LID RETRACTION

Lower lid retraction is defined as the inferior malposition of the lower eyelid margin without eyelid eversion or inversion. The cause of lower eyelid retraction can be multifactorial. Typically, instability of the lower eyelid is caused by horizontal laxity involving the tarsoligamentous sling or the orbicularis muscle. Other causes of lower lid retraction can involve scarred or tethered middle lamellae due to prior surgery or trauma and weakened vertical support of the lower lid due to midface descent. Orbital proptosis is another common cause of lower eyelid retraction, which may be due to thyroid exophthalmopathy or nonthyroid causes.

Lateral Canthal Tendon Laxity

Lower lid retraction due to lateral canthal tendon laxity is the simplest problem to fix of potential pathologies that contribute to lower lid malposition. Causes of lateral canthal tendon laxity include senile or paralytic laxity, congenital, traumatic, and/or iatrogenic. Lateral canthal tendon laxity can be determined by placing a finger over the lateral canthal angle and directing the force in a superior and lateral direction. This action will mimic a lateral canthal tendon tightening procedure; if the central lid position is appropriately positioned along the inferior aspect of the limbus, this may be the only procedure necessary for correction of the malposition. Usually, patients with minimal to moderate lid retraction can be corrected with solely a lateral canthoplasty procedure; however, moderate to severe cases will require adjunctive procedures.

Various techniques have been described for lower lid tightening in an effort to prevent or treat lateral canthal tendon laxity.[7–13] The tarsal strip procedure is a commonly performed and popular procedure for lateral canthal tendon tightening[7,13] (Fig. 2). Careful attention should be given to reestablishing the lateral canthal angle with a suture reapproximating the gray line of the upper and lower lids to prevent any postoperative blunting.

Middle Lamella Scarring

Middle lamella scarring refers to fibrosis between the orbital septum and the capsulopalpebral fascia or lower eyelid retractors. This scarring can occur iatrogenically or traumatically due to disruption of the orbital septum resulting in contracture.[6] The septum naturally inserts anteriorly to the capsulopalpebral fascia roughly 5 mm inferior to the tarsus; however, contracture and disruption of the septum can lead to fusion of the 2 layers (Fig. 3A). Patipa[6] posits the fusion can occur because of inflammation of the orbital fat pads. This scar band can lead to a more hollowed eye appearance by posterior displacement of the orbital fat pads. This displacement will ultimately retract the lower lid inferiorly oftentimes resulting in scleral show. A vertical traction test, which involves pushing the lower eyelid upward over the cornea with the examiner's finger, can help establish the diagnosis if there is resistance to movement suggesting middle lamella scarring.[2]

The goal for treatment of middle lamella scarring is to release the capsulopalpebral fascia from the scarred orbital septum. Through a transconjunctival approach, the conjunctiva and capsulopalpebral fascia are released from the inferior tarsal margin. The plane between the capsulopalpebral fascia and the orbital septum is then released of scar tissue, which will allow the orbital fat to resume its natural position between the two

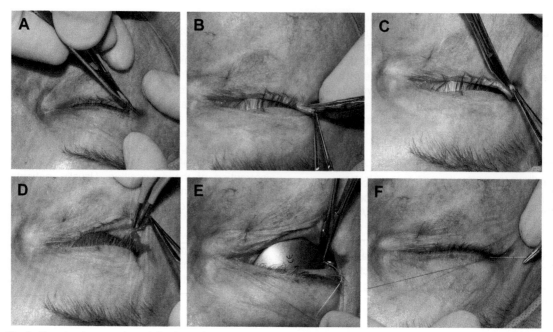

Fig. 2. Tarsal strip procedure: (*A*) A lateral canthotomy is made down to the periosteum of the lateral orbital rim followed by a (*B*) cantholysis of the inferior limb of the lateral canthal tendon. (*C*) The gray line and anterior lamella is then dissected free, and the tightly adherent conjunctiva is scraped or (*D*) cauterized off the posterior aspect of the tarsus. The tarsus is then shortened accordingly and (*E*) resuspended at the Whitnall tubercle with a suture anchored to the periosteum of the medial rim of the lateral orbit. (*F*) The excess skin and muscle may be trimmed away, and the skin is closed with absorbable suture. (*Courtesy of* Steven Couch, MD, St Louis, MO.)

lamellae.[6] A spacer graft is then harvested and thinned to the thickness of the tarsus. The spacer graft is then placed between the inferior tarsal edge and the recessed conjunctiva and capsulopalpebral fascia (see **Fig. 3**B). The spacer graft allows for restoration of lower lid retractor height and supports the lower eyelid following release of the scarred tissue. Spacer grafts can

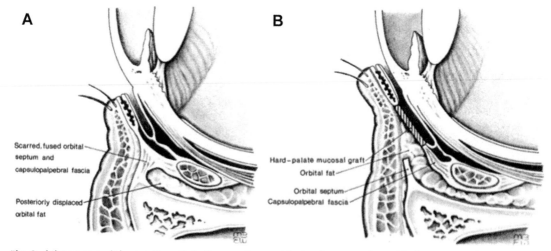

Fig. 3. (*A*) Lower eyelid retraction. Note the scarring and fusion between the orbital septum and capsulopalpebral fascia, which results in lower eyelid retraction and posterior displacement of the orbital fat. This displacement contributes to the hollow-eyed appearance in these patients after cosmetic surgery. (*B*) Capsulopalpebral fascia released from inferior tarsus and recessed, the inserted hard palate/mucosal graft spacer, and the released, scarred orbital septum. This release allows the orbital fat to return to its normal anatomic plane. (*From* Patipa M. The evaluation and management of lower eyelid retraction following cosmetic surgery. Plast Reconstr Surg 2000;106(2):439, 444; with permission.)

be autogenous tissue, including hard palate, temporalis fascia, dermis, auricular cartilage, septal cartilage, tarsal grafts, or alloplastic implants, such as acellular dermis (AlloDerm, LifeCell Corporation, Bridgewater, NJ).[14–20] The hard palate graft remains the gold standard because it most closely resembles the tarsus in consistency and structural integrity and exhibits predictable outcomes compared with other autogenous or alloplastic options. An excellent, detailed description of this technique can be further viewed in the article by Patipa.[6] Usually, this procedure is performed in conjunction with a lateral canthal tendon tightening procedure.

Midface Descent

Midface descent occurs with aging due to gravitational forces and morphologic changes. Potential findings of malar decent include the presence of a distinct lid-cheek interface, hollowed appearance in the infraorbital region, and an inferiorly displaced malar fat pad along with a flat malar eminence.[21] The loss of bony and soft tissue support of the lower eyelid can result in malposition of the lower lid. The treatment of the midfacial tissues may be necessary in certain cases of lower lid retraction where lateral canthal tightening or spacer treatment have not fully addressed the malposition. Repositioning of the suborbicularis oculi fat and malar fat pad can be performed through supraperiosteal or subperiosteal midface elevation techniques. Approaches to the midface have been described, including a transconjunctival, transtemporal, and subciliary approaches.[22–24] Additional treatments to augment this region can include fat transfer, filler, and placement of malar implants; however, the exact role and their potential to prevent or correct lower lid retraction, particularly in negative vector eyelids, has not been fully studied.[25] It is thought that suspension or support of the malar region can facilitate recruitment of new skin to the lower eyelid, providing less distraction at the external lamellar plane.[2,23,26]

ECTROPION

Ectropion is the eversion of the eyelid margin often in conjunction with lid retraction. Ectropion may be categorized as involutional, cicatricial, paralytic, or mechanical. Ectropion can present with epiphora from punctal eversion and conjunctival irritation and keratitis due to lagophthalmos. These symptoms can be distressing to patients and result in long-term ocular complications.

Involutional Ectropion

Involutional ectropion is the most common form of ectropion encountered and is due to horizontal lower lid laxity secondary to age-related weakening of the canthal ligaments and orbicularis muscle. Patients with involutional ectropion have been found to have larger-than-average tarsal plates for their age with normal or decreased tone of the pretarsal/preseptal orbicularis muscle in conjunction with increased laxity of the tarsoligamentous sling.[27] Additional age-related descent of malar fat pad and midface volume loss contributes to the loss of support of the lower lid. Treatment of involutional ectropion invariably requires correction of lower lid laxity through horizontal tightening of the lower eyelid. This treatment is most commonly performed through a lateral tarsal strip procedure (**Fig. 4**); but depending on the functional needs and aesthetic concerns, other horizontal tightening procedures, including lateral canthopexy, pentagonal wedge resection, and inferior or lateral retinacular canthoplasty, may be performed.[7,11,28,29] In cases of medial involutional ectropion, patients may present with epiphora due to punctal eversion. A medial conjunctival spindle procedure can be performed to reoppose the lower lid to the globe. This procedure is done by excising an ellipse of medial conjunctiva and lower lid retractors and shortening the medial posterior lamella (see **Fig. 4**).

Cicatricial Ectropion

Cicatricial ectropion is due to vertical shortening of the anterior or middle lamella most often due to scarring of the lower lid skin following a lower lid injury or inflammatory process. Deficiency of the anterior lamella following excessive skin and/or muscle removal following a transcutaneous lower lid blepharoplasty has been a known cause of cicatricial ectropion.[30,31] Transconjunctival blepharoplasty has a significantly lower risk of ectropion, even with excision of lower eyelid skin.[32] Inadvertent suturing of the orbital septum can also result in scar fixation of the lower lid. Excessive orbital fat removal or postoperative hematoma resulting in fat necrosis has also been linked to postblepharoplasty ectropion.[33]

A graded approach should be taken to manage cicatricial ectropion. If the ectropion is noted early in the postoperative period, nonsurgical interventions may be used to mitigate the lower lid retraction and eversion with conservative vertical traction and massaging of the lower eyelid. Prolonged or significant conjunctival chemosis producing downward pressure on the lower eyelid can be treated with topical lubricants and

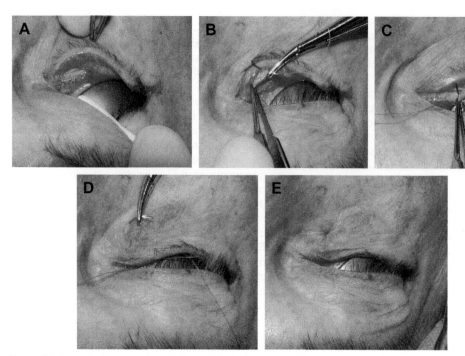

Fig. 4. Medial spindle procedure: (*A*) An elliptical excision of conjunctiva and lower lid retractor is performed. (*B–D*) The defect is closed with buried transcutaneous mattress suture (5–0 chromic gut) resulting in (*E*) inversion of the medial lid margin. (*Courtesy of* Steven Couch, MD, St Louis, MO.)

antiinflammatory ophthalmic medication to prevent scarring in a retracted position. Persistent or significant ectropion will require secondary surgical intervention to correct the problem. Anterior lamellar shortening due to over resection of skin or scar contracture most often requires treatment with full-thickness skin graft in combination with a horizontal lid-tightening procedure to lengthen the lower lid height (**Fig. 5**). The upper eyelid skin offers the ideal match for grafting; however, if unavailable because of prior upper lid blepharoplasty, other donor sites may include postauricular or supraclavicular skin. Ectropion due to scar contracture of the orbital septum or adhesion of the middle lamella to the inferior orbital rim will require a transconjunctival release of the cicatrix and correction of the deficient middle lamella with spacer grafts as mentioned earlier. Often times, the causes of cicatricial ectropion can be multifactorial and may require adjunctive procedures, including lower lid volume augmentation and midface lifting techniques, to support the lower eyelid to oppose the downward forces on the lower eyelid.[34–36]

Paralytic Ectropion

Paralytic ectropion can be seen because of loss of orbicularis muscle tone following facial nerve paralysis. Concomitant upper eyelid lagophthalmos

is usually present because of the paralytic upper lid orbicularis dysfunction. In cases of temporary facial paralysis, eye care with lubricating drops and eyelid taping may be sufficient to manage any ectropion. However, prolonged or permanent paralysis will require surgical intervention to treat the ectropion. Horizontal lid tightening procedures are usually indicated and may require both medial and lateral canthoplasties. Fascia lata or silicone suspension sling may be required to support the ectropic lower lid in conjunction with release of the lower lid retractors and placement of spacer grafts. Medial and lateral tarsorrhaphies may be required for patients with recalcitrant corneal disease.

Mechanical Ectropion

Mechanical ectropion occurs because of a mass or conjunctival edema near the lid margin physically displacing the lower lid. The management of mechanical ectropion is specific to the disease process and is aimed at eliminating the downward and everting vectors of force on the lower eyelid.

ENTROPION

Entropion is lower lid malposition characterized by the inward rotation of the eyelid margin. The causes of entropion are multifactorial and can be

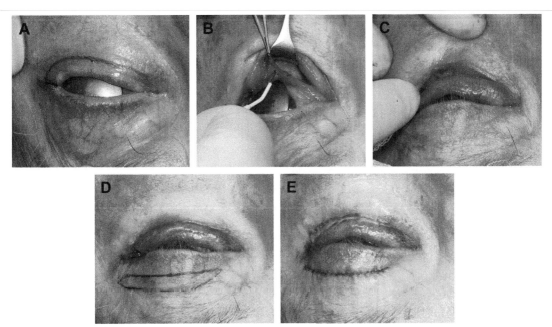

Fig. 5. Full-thickness skin graft (FTSG) repair of cicatricial ectropion: (*A*) Incision for lateral canthotomy and subtarsal release is marked. (*B*) After lateral canthotomy and cantholysis is performed, a transconjunctival incision is made just inferior to the tarsal plate and a segment of conjunctiva and lower lid retractors is removed to allow the lower lid to intorsion. (*C*) A subtarsal incision is made with care taken to avoid injuring the orbicularis muscle. The posterior lamella is then closed with buried mattress sutures. (*D*) An appropriately sized graft is marked and harvested for FTSG of the lower lid (ideally from the upper eyelid). (*E*) Repair following placement of the FTSG and horizontal lid tightening via tarsal strip procedure. (*Courtesy of* Steven Couch, MD, St Louis, MO.)

congenital or acquired. Congenital entropion is extremely rare and usually requires early surgical intervention to avoid ocular complication.

Involutional Entropion

Involutional entropion is the most common form of acquired entropion and is due to horizontal lid laxity and dehiscence of the lower lid retractors in conjunction with a normal or hyperactive preseptal orbicularis that overrides a smaller-than-average tarsal plate.[27] Additionally, involutional enophthalmos can contribute to lower lid inversion. Preoperative assessment of the lower lid will likely show increased lower lid laxity with easy eversion of the lower lid inferior traction. The lower lid margin usually remains in a neutral position following inferior traction until patients blink. In mild cases, nonsurgical treatment of involutional entropion with botulinum toxin of the orbicularis has been proposed.[37,38] Surgical techniques for correction of involutional entropion are aimed at reducing horizontal lid laxity and reinsertion of the lower lid retractors to the inferior border of the tarsal plate or the anterior lamella at the level of the tarsal plate to reduce upward movement of the preseptal orbicularis muscle.[39,40] For temporary treatment of entropion, an everting suture technique has been described by Quickert and Rathbun,[41] which consists of multiple horizontal mattress sutures placed from the conjunctival fornix through the lower lid skin below the lash line.[11]

Cicatricial Entropion

Cicatricial entropion results from a vertically shortened posterior lamella, usually from scarring of the conjunctiva or tarsus. Common conditions that may contribute to cicatricial entropion include transconjunctival approach for orbital or periorbital surgery, trauma, chemical burns, conjunctival infections or inflammation (eg, ocular cicatricial pemphigoid, Stevens-Johnson syndrome). The cause of the cicatricial entropion should be identified before any attempted surgical correction. Systemic inflammatory conditions may require urgent initiation of treatment before surgery. Examination of the lower lid may reveal tarsal fibrosis with blunting and shortening of the conjunctival fornices and symblepharon causing a tethered lower lid that resists downward retraction and eversion. The goals of surgical treatment include anterior rotation of the lid margin, repositioning the lashes away from the cornea, and restoration of the posterior lamellar height. The placement of mucosal spacer grafts (eg, hard palate mucosa) via a transconjunctival approach following scar lysis has been widely supported for the treatment of cicatricial entropion.[42,43] Additional surgical procedures have also been described, including tarsal fracture, blepharotomy, and suturing techniques.[44–46]

Spastic Entropion

Spastic entropion occurs because of excessive contraction of the orbicularis muscle with override of the preseptal orbicularis muscle over the tarsal plate. This complication can occur with blepharospasms or hemifacial spasms and is associated with ocular irritation or inflammation. Spastic entropion may be temporary and intermittent and can be effectively treated with paralyzing the offending orbicularis muscle with botulinum toxin or suture eversion of the lower lid.[47]

SUMMARY

There are many causes of lower lid malposition ranging from rare instances of congenital causes to more commonly encountered effects of gravity and aging and iatrogenic complications. Intricate knowledge of the trilamellar anatomy along with the supportive structures of the lower eyelid and midface will help direct surgical and nonsurgical techniques for correction of the lower lid malposition. In many instances, horizontal lid laxity plays a crucial role in lower lid malpositioning. Surgeons need to be able to preoperatively assess lower lid tone and support and be facile with horizontal lid-tightening procedures to prevent any untoward postoperative results. Deficiencies or restrictions of one or more lamellae requires autogenous or alloplastic grafting to restore vertical height and mobility. Adjunctive procedures may be considered to support the lower lid, such as midface lifting to restore malar fat pad positioning or hyaluronic acid augmentation of the lower lid.

ACKNOWLEDGMENT

The authors would like to acknowledge Dr Steven Couch, oculoplastic and reconstructive surgeon at Washington University in St Louis for his photographs.

REFERENCES

1. Branham G, Holds JB. Brow-upper lid anatomy, aging and aesthetic analysis. Facial Plast Surg Clin North Am 2015;23(2):117–27.
2. Patel MP, Shapiro MD, Spinelli HM. Combined hard palate spacer graft, midface suspension, and lateral canthoplasty for lower eyelid retraction: a tripartite approach. Plast Reconstr Surg 2005;115:2105–14.
3. Owsley JQ. Lifting the malar fat pad for correction of prominent nasolabial folds. Plast Reconstr Surg 1993;91:463.
4. Jelks GW, Jelks EB. The influence of orbital and eyelid anatomy on the palpebral aperture. Clin Plast Surg 1991;18:183–95.
5. Wolfe SA, Kearney R. Blepharoplasty in the patient with exophthalmos. Clin Plast Surg 1993;20:275–83.
6. Patipa M. The evaluation and management of lower eyelid retraction following cosmetic surgery. Plast Reconstr Surg 2000;106(2):438–53.
7. Anderson RL, Gordy DD. The tarsal strip procedure. Arch Ophthalmol 1979;97:2192–6.
8. Ousterhout DK, Weil RB. The role of the lateral canthal tendon in lower eyelid laxity. Plast Reconstr Surg 1982;69:620.
9. Rees TD. Prevention of ectropion by horizontal shortening of the lower lid during blepharoplasty. Ann Plast Surg 1983;11:17.
10. Flowers RS. Canthopexy as a routine blepharoplasty component. Clin Plast Surg 1993;20:351.
11. Lisman RD, Campbell J. Tarsal suspension canthoplasty. Aesthetic Surg J 1999;19:412.
12. Carraway JH. The role of canthoplasty in aesthetic blepharoplasty. Aesthetic Surg J 1998;18:277.
13. Della Roca DA. The lateral tarsal strip: illustrated pearls. Facial Plast Surg 2007;3:200–2.
14. Marks MW, Argenta LC, Friedman RJ, et al. Conchal cartilage and composite grafts for correction of lower lid retraction. Plast Reconstr Surg 1989; 83:629.
15. Wearne MJ, Sandy C, Rose GE, et al. Autogenous hard palate mucosa: the ideal lower eyelid spacer? Br J Ophthalmol 2001;85:1183.
16. Kersten RC, Kulwin DR, Levartovsky S, et al. Management of lower lid retraction with hard palate mucosa graft. Arch Ophthalmol 1990;108:1339.
17. Hurwitz JJ, Archer KF, Gruss JS. Treatment of severe lower eyelid retraction with scleral and free skin grafts and bipedicle orbicularis flap. Ophthalmic Surg 1990;21:167.
18. Morton AD, Nelson C, Ikada Y, et al. Porous polyethylene as a spacer graft in the treatment of lower eyelid retraction. Ophthal Plast Reconstr Surg 2000;16:146.
19. Cohen MS, Shorr N. Eyelid reconstruction with hard palate mucosa graft. Ophthal Plast Reconstr Surg 1992;8:183.
20. Taban M, Douglas R, Li T, et al. Efficacy of thick acellular human dermis for lower eyelid reconstruction: comparison with hard palate and thin AlloDerm grafts. Arch Facial Plast Surg 2005;7(1):38–44.
21. McCord CD, Codner MA, Hester TR. Redraping the inferior orbicularis arc. Plast Reconstr Surg 1998; 102:2471.

22. Anderson RD, Lo MW. Endoscopic malar-midface suspension procedure. Plast Reconstr Surg 1998; 102:2196.

23. Hinderer UT. Vertical preperiosteal rejuvenation of the frame of the eyelids and midface. Plast Reconstr Surg 1999;104:1482.

24. Marshak H, Morrow DM, Dresner SC. Small incision preperiosteal midface lift for correction of lower eyelid retraction. Ophthal Plast Reconstr Surg 2010;26:176–81.

25. Le PT, Peckinpaugh J, Naficy S, et al. Effect of autologous fat injection on lower eyelid position. Ophthal Plast Reconstr Surg 2014;30:504–7.

26. Hester TR Jr, Codner MA, McCord CD, et al. Evolution of technique of the direct transblepharoplasty approach for the correction of lower lid and midfacial aging: maximizing results and minimizing complications in a 5-year experience. Plast Reconstr Surg 2000;105(1):393–406; discussion 407–8.

27. Bashour M, Harvey J. Causes of involutional ectropion and entropion – age-related tarsal changes are the key. Ophthal Plast Reconstr Surg 2000; 16(2):131–41.

28. Fagien S. Algorithm for canthoplasty: the lateral retinacular suspension: a simplified suture canthopexy. Plast Reconstr Surg 1999;103:2042.

29. Jelks GW, Glat PM, Jelks EB, et al. The inferior retinacular lateral canthoplasty: a new technique. Plast Reconstr Surg 1997;100:1262.

30. Friedman WH. Ectropion after blepharoplasty: experimental and clinical observations. Arch Otolaryngol Head Neck Surg 1979;105:455–60.

31. McGraw BL, Adamson PA. Postblepharoplasty ectropion. Arch Otolaryngol Head Neck Surg 1991; 117:852–6.

32. Rosenberg DB, Lattman J, Shah AR. Prevention of lower eyelid malposition after blepharoplasty. Arch Facial Plast Surg 2007;9(6):434–8.

33. Edgarton MT. Causes and prevention of lower lid ectropion following blepharoplasty. Plast Reconstr Surg 1972;49:367–73.

34. Jacono AA, Stong BC. Combined transconjunctival release and midface-lift for postblepharoplasty

35. Fezza JP. Nonsurgical treatment of cicatricial ectropion with hyaluronic acid fuller. Plast Reconstr Surg 2008;121(3):1009–14.

36. Chung JE, Yen MT. Midface lifting as an adjunct procedure in ectropion repair. Ann Plast Surg 2007; 59(6):635–40.

37. Steel DH, Hoh HB, Harrad RA, et al. Botulinum toxin for the temporary treatment of involutional lower lid entropion: a clinical and morphological study. Eye 1997;11:472–5.

38. Clarke JR, Spalton DJ. Treatment of senile entropion with botulinum toxin. Br J Ophthalmol 1988; 72:361–2.

39. Schaefer AJ. Variation in the pathophysiology of involutional entropion and its treatment. Ophthalmic Surg 1983;14:653–5.

40. Wies FA. Surgical treatment of entropion. J Int Coll Surg 1954;21:758–60.

41. Quickert MH, Rathbun E. Suture repair of entropion. Arch Ophthalmol 1971;85:304–5.

42. Bartley GB, Kay PP. Posterior lamellar eyelid reconstruction with a hard palate mucosal graft. Am J Ophthalmol 1989;107:609–12.

43. Baylis HI, Hamako C. Tarsal grafting for correction of cicatricial entropion. Ophthalmic Surg 1979;10:42–8.

44. Millman AL, Katzen LB, Putterman AM. Cicatricial entropion: an analysis of its treatment with transverse blepharotomy and marginal rotation. Ophthalmic Surg 1989;20:575–9.

45. Wojno TH. Lid splitting with lash resection for cicatricial entropion and trichiasis. Ophthal Plast Reconstr Surg 1992;8:287–9.

46. Sodhi PK, Yadava U, Mehta DK. Efficacy of lamellar division for correcting cicatricial lid entropion and its associated features unrectified by the tarsal fracture technique. Orbit 2002;21(1):9–17.

47. Elston JS, Russell RWR. Effect of treatment with botulinum toxin on neurogenic blepharospasm. Br Med J 1985;209:1857–9.

Upper Eyelid Reconstruction

Gabriela Mabel Espinoza, MD*, Angela Michelle Prost, FNP-BC

KEYWORDS

- Upper eyelid ● Reconstruction ● Surgical techniques ● Eyelid defect ● Skin graft
- Myocutaneous flap

KEY POINTS

- In eyelid wound closure, tension should be drawn horizontally to avoid ectropion or lid retraction.
- Local myocutaneous advancement flaps may be used for smaller defects. For moderate to large defects, the Tenzel semicircular advancement flap technique or the Cutler-Beard 2-staged procedure may be used, respectively.
- When the lid margin is involved, eyelash growth may be compromised. Loss of the medial eyelid margin is further complicated by the lacrimal drainage system and medial canthal tendon attachment to the lacrimal crest.
- Understanding the factors of upper eyelid reconstruction and knowing different techniques for repair prepare the surgeon to create a functional and cosmetically acceptable eyelid.

INTRODUCTION

A patient undergoing reconstructive surgery of the eyelids desires results that best restore the eyelid function while optimizing the aesthetic outcome. Reconstruction of the upper eyelid is more challenging than that of the lower eyelid due to the highly specialized function of the upper eyelid. The eyelid is a thin structure with the ability to open and close to lubricate and protect the ocular surface while allowing an unobscured visual axis to see. The maintenance of the corneal surface is critical for sharp vision and patient comfort. Any disruption of the eyelid tissue can cause loss of mobility of the eyelid by scarring and tethering of the lid margin. Loss of tissue is particularly troublesome because the eyelid must maintain its mobility, flexibility, function, and a good mucosal surface to be in contact with the sensitive cornea. Dynamic blink and range of movement is often at odds with the need to replace tissue to allow for

the eyelid to close. Inability to close the eyelids together can cause drying of the eye, which leads to blurred vision, light sensitivity, and increased risk of infection that could eventually lead to loss of the eye. Multiple surgeries may be required to achieve the desired results, to address first the loss of tissue and then the loss of function. In addition, the surgeon must also take into consideration the appearance of the eyelid, which can have an adverse impact on a patient's quality of life.

Defects of the upper eyelid may be related to various causes, including but not limited to congenital defects and traumatic injury, or follow oncologic resection. The type of reconstruction depends on the anatomic deficits identified, including the vertical, horizontal, and depth dimensions as well as the availability of regional and distant tissue for reconstruction. This article focuses on reconstruction techniques used in the correction of eyelid defects that involve loss of tissue.

Disclosure Statement: The authors have nothing to disclose.
Department of Ophthalmology, Saint Louis University Eye Institute, Saint Louis University School of Medicine, 1755 South Grand Boulevard, St Louis, MO 63104, USA
* Corresponding author.
E-mail address: gespinoz@slu.edu

Facial Plast Surg Clin N Am 24 (2016) 173–182
http://dx.doi.org/10.1016/j.fsc.2015.12.007

ANTERIOR LAMELLAR UPPER EYELID DEFECTS

The anterior lamella of the eyelid includes skin and orbicularis oculi muscle. Small defects less than 1 cm in diameter can heal well by secondary intention if they are superficial and favorably located in the medial canthus, which has bony support, or along the pretarsal skin, in which the tarsus lends support to the wound. Contracture of the wound is typically noted by 2 to 6 weeks, at which time the need for further surgery can be determined for possible sequelae, such as lid retraction or ectropion of the eyelid margin.[1,2]

When there is redundant skin adjacent to the defect, primary closure is often possible with or without undermining the skin. The ability to close without a formal flap depends on the quality of the skin and the amount of redundancy present. Closure should draw the tension horizontally to avoid ectropion or lid retraction, although aligning scars with the lid crease can help camouflage the scar.[3,4]

When more tissue recruitment is needed, local myocutaneous advancement flaps are the preferred choice because they provide optimal color and texture match, near-normal innervation, minimal contracture, and a rich blood supply. The most useful flaps in this area include rhombic, transposition, and advancement flaps (**Fig. 1**).

When the lid margin is involved, the anterior lamella contains eyelashes, which may be lost or may regrow through scar tissue, causing trichiasis. Special consideration should be made if the eyelashes are involved because this marginal tissue is adherent to the underlying tarsus and does not allow for direct closure. The upper eyelid eyelashes are more visible than the lower eyelid lashes and maintaining a continuous lash line can be an important part of the final cosmesis. Converting this defect into a full-thickness defect can be a viable and preferred option when there is less than 33% of the lash margin loss. The lack of lashes laterally is not as noticeable because it is centrally and there seems to be a compensatory eyelash follicle mechanism that maintains the total number of eyelashes.[5]

Skin grafts offer replacement of the eyelid skin with tissue taken from a distant source when local options are exhausted. A full-thickness skin graft is preferable to a split-thickness skin graft due to less wound contracture. Optimal donor sites have thin dermis, minimal hair, and similar color and texture to the eyelid. Contralateral upper eyelid skin is the best match, followed by lower eyelid skin, preauricular or postauricular skin, supraclavicular skin, and inner upper arm skin.

The color match from these sites has been found to be good in 85% to 94% of patients, with more hypopigmentation noted more from supraclavicular and inner upper arm donor sites.[6,7] Complications of periocular full-thickness skin grafts occur in approximately 12% of cases.[8] The most common complications were hypertrophy (42.3%), partial graft failure (27.2%) and wound contraction (15.3%).

A split-thickness graft allows for significantly more coverage of a wound because the donor site heals by secondary intent and the hair-bearing skin may be used as the follicles are left behind. The contracture of a split-thickness graft can cause eyelid retraction and compensatory eyelid tightening or a temporary tarsorrhaphy may be needed to reduce this effect during the healing phase. Massage, steroid ointment or injections, and silicone gel application can also be useful in the postoperative phase to improve hypertrophy or contracture of the skin grafts.

FULL-THICKNESS UPPER EYELID DEFECTS
Canthal Defects

Loss of the medial eyelid margin is complicated by the presence of the lacrimal drainage system and the medial canthal tendon attachment to the anterior and posterior lacrimal crest. Reconstruction of the lacrimal drainage system typically involves silicone stent intubation of the remaining canalicular system to maintain patency. Although the upper eyelid is not as critical in tear drainage as the lower eyelid is, delayed repair can be difficult to achieve with excellent success rate of primary repair.[9]

Identifying a suitable anchoring point for the medial upper eyelid is important for stabilization of the lid margin. Optimal choices include the stump of the medial canthal tendon or the periosteum of the medial orbital wall. Microplates, miniplates, resorbable and nonresorbable screws, and transnasal wiring have been used when insufficient soft tissue remains.[10–12]

Loss of the lateral canthal tendon may be replaced by creating a lateral tarsal strip or a periosteal flap from the lateral orbital rim.[13,14] It is best to create an oblique strip of periosteum hinged at the orbital rim that is longer than believed needed. The lateral orbital rim provides the ability to drill a full thickness hole for direct anchoring to the bone with suture or wires if there is not enough soft tissue.[3,14]

Small Defects

Depending on the laxity of the eyelid tissues, full-thickness defects of the lid margin involving up to one-third of the horizontal length may be closed

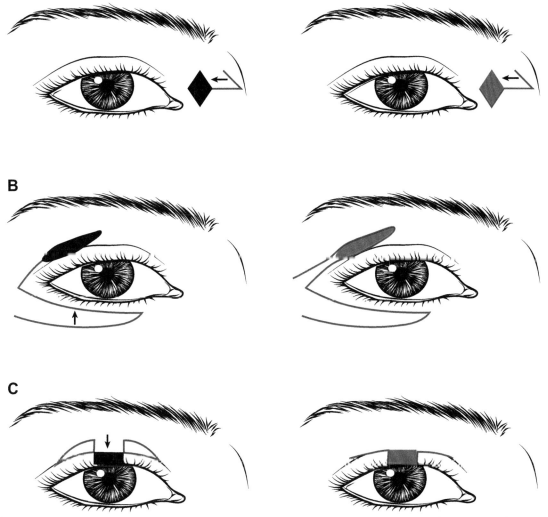

Fig. 1. Periocular flaps. (*A*) Skin defect in black on the left, arrow showing rhombic skin flap to rotate laterally and cover the defect (grey on the right) with primary closure of the donor site. (*B*) Skin defect in black on the left parallel to the eyelid margin, arrow showing transposition skin flap to rotate superiorly and cover the defect (grey on the right) with primary closure of the donor site. (*C*) Pretarsal skin defect in black on the left, arrow showing supratarsal skin to be advanced and cover the defect (grey on the right). Lateral excess of skin removed to close the donor site without redundancy.

with direct closure. Assessment includes pulling the edges of the defect together to confirm the wound is not under too much tension. Minimal tension can be released with a lateral canthotomy or cantholysis. If superior tarsus remains, completion of a pentagonal resection or complete excision of the residual tarsus may be performed to allow for the ends to meet appropriately. If there is minimal tarsal loss with good skin laxity, then a local tarso-conjunctival flap may be used to recreate the posterior lamella with skin or myocutaneous advancement flap. Approximately 4 mm of vertical height in the residual tarsus is needed to maintain stability of the lid margin. As discussed previously,

the loss of eyelashes can be aesthetically displeasing but preferable if tissue recruitment from the lateral canthal angle is difficult.

The steps of eyelid margin repair include

1. Reforming the lid margin: use a 5-0 or 6-0 Vicryl suture on a spatulated needle to place partial-thickness pass through the tarsus. Properly align the lid margin by positioning the suture obliquely through the tarsus with the anterior pass level with the base of the eyelashes and the posterior pass level with the corner of the lid margin. Maintain partial-thickness passes to avoid corneal abrasion (**Fig. 2**A).

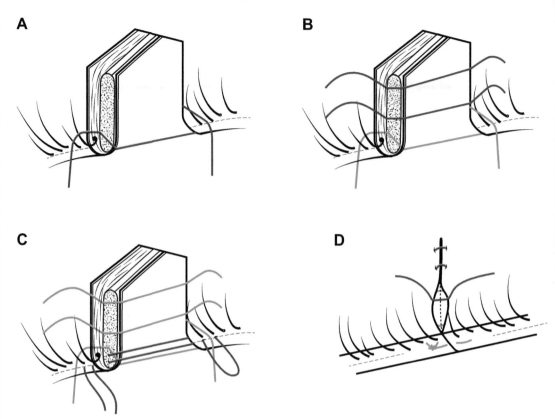

Fig. 2. Lid margin repair. (*A*) Align the lid margin using a 5-0 Vicryl suture diagonally through the tarsus. (*B*) Suture the superior tarsal plate for stabilization. (*C*) Evert the marginal wound edge with a 7-0 Vicryl suture in a vertical mattress fashion. (*D*) Close the overlying skin.

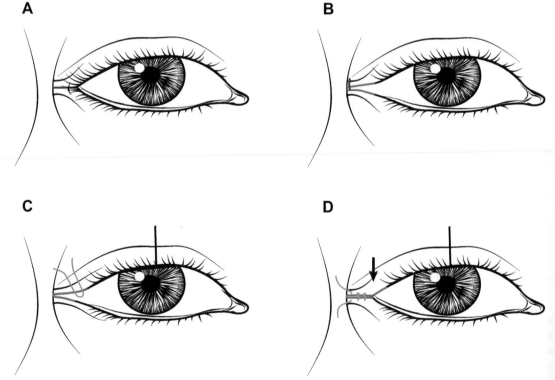

Fig. 3. Lateral canthotomy and cantholysis. (*A*) Open the lateral canthus with a full-thickness incision down to the orbital rim. (*B*) Transect the superior crus of the lateral canthal tendon. (*C*) After repairing the eyelid defect, recreate the lateral eyelid margin with a 7-0 Vicryl suture in a full-thickness horizontal mattress fashion. (*D*) Close the lateral canthal skin.

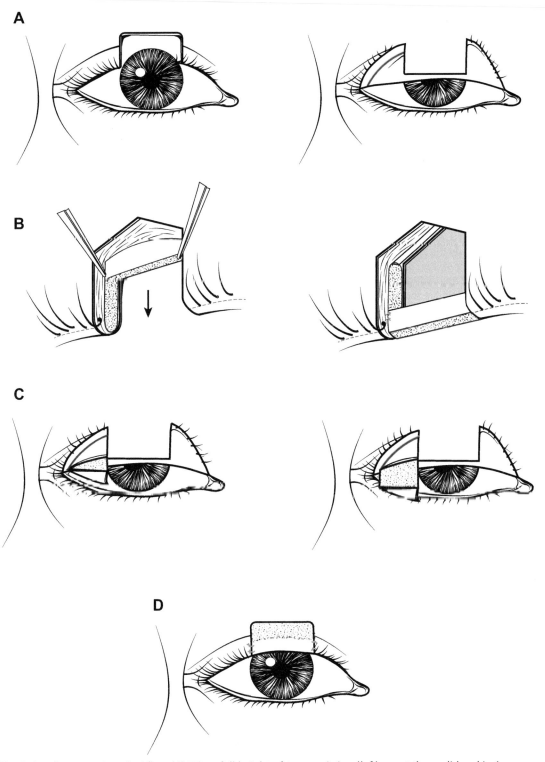

Fig. 4. Local tarsoconjunctival flap. (*A*) When full height of tarsus missing (*left*), evert the eyelid and incise superior tarsus of remaining eyelid (*right*) leaving behind a 4-mm margin for stability. (*B*) When at least 4 mm of superior tarsus remains in a full-thickness defect (*left*), advance the remaining tarsus to the margin (*right*). (*C*) Create a tarsoconjunctival flap by dissecting the anterior tissue off the flap (*left*) and create relaxing incisions in the conjunctiva superiorly (*right*). (*D*) Transpose the tarsoconjunctival flap into the defect to reform the margin.

2. Closure of the tarsal plate: use interrupted 5-0 or 6-0 Vicryl suture to place interrupted partial-thickness passes along the superior aspect of the tarsus (**Fig. 2**B).
3. Everting the lid margin to prevent notching: place a 7-0 Vicryl suture in a vertical mattress fashion at the gray line of the lid margin. This suture can be cut short and left to absorb (**Fig. 2**C).
4. Closing the skin: the tension on the skin should be reduced with the closure of the tarsal plate. Interrupted or running suture may be used to close the skin (**Fig. 2**D).

The steps of canthotomy and cantholysis include

1. Canthotomy: use Westcott scissors to open the lateral canthus the length of the inferior tarsus, stopping where the conjunctiva is no longer adherent to the tarsus. Identify the canthal tendon and split the tendon down to the orbital rim (**Fig. 3**A).
2. Cantholysis: place the eyelid under tension by distracting the eyelid away from the globe. Visualize and feel the canthal tendon attachment to the periosteum by strumming the tissue with the Westcott scissors. Transect the superior crus of the tendon as close to the

periosteum as possible by turning the scissors 90° to the eyelid margin and pushing it against the lateral orbital rim while cutting (**Fig. 3**B).
3. Closing the eyelid margin defect, as described previously.
4. Placing a 7-0 Vicryl mattress suture through the advanced edge of skin full thickness through orbicularis muscle fibers, the tendon, and the conjunctival edge to lend support and thickness to the newly formed lid margin (**Fig. 3**C).
5. Closing the canthotomy (**Fig. 3**D).

The steps of a local tarsoconjunctival flap include

1. Everting the remaining eyelid tarsus and create an incision parallel to and 4 mm superior to the lid margin (**Fig. 4**A). If there is a central full-thickness defect with remaining superior tarsus in the wound, then it may be directly advanced to the lid margin (**Fig. 4**B).
2. Dissecting away the overlying levator aponeurosis and Müller muscle up to the superior fornix, leaving the conjunctiva attached to the tarsus. Create relaxing incisions in the conjunctiva to allow transposition into the wound (**Fig. 4**C).
3. Suturing the edges of the tarsus to the marginal tarsus (**Fig. 4**D).

A

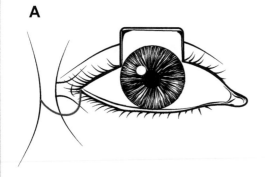

B

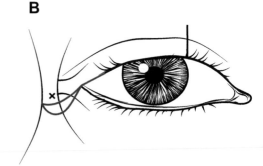

C

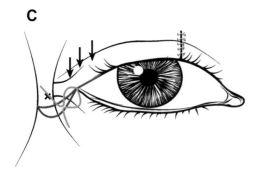

D

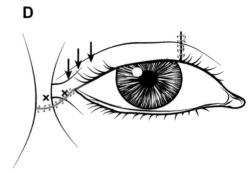

Fig. 5. Tenzel semicircular advancement flap. (*A*) Mark out the lateral semicircular flap to recruit as much skin as needed. (*B*) Create the flap and undermine until the wound edges can be opposed easily. Anchor the flap by fixating orbicularis layer to the underlying periosteum at the level of insertion of the inferior canthal tendon. (*C*) Reform the lateral canthal angle with a 7-0 Vicryl suture attaching the orbicularis layer to the inferior canthal tendon. (*D*) Close the lateral canthal skin.

Moderate Defects

Repairing larger defects of the eyelid requires critical evaluation of the surrounding tissues. Direct closure of a wound affecting one-third to two-thirds of the eyelid may be done if there is enough horizontal laxity of the eyelid. If the wound is too tight, then consider a canthotomy and cantholysis. If the temporal skin can be mobilized, then move to a semicircular advancement (Tenzel) flap technique.[3,15] If the lateral canthus has been lost, then a local tarsoconjunctival flap may be used along with a periosteal strip. The anterior lamella could then be replaced with a full-thickness skin graft or myocutaneous flap. If there is enough anterior lamella to support a graft, then alternatives may be used to recreate the posterior lamella, such as a free tarsal graft from the contralateral upper eyelid, hard palate, or mucosa-lined acellular dermis.[16–18] Myocutaneous flaps would supply the blood supply for these grafts which lend support to the lid margin.

The steps of a semicircular advancement (Tenzel) flap include

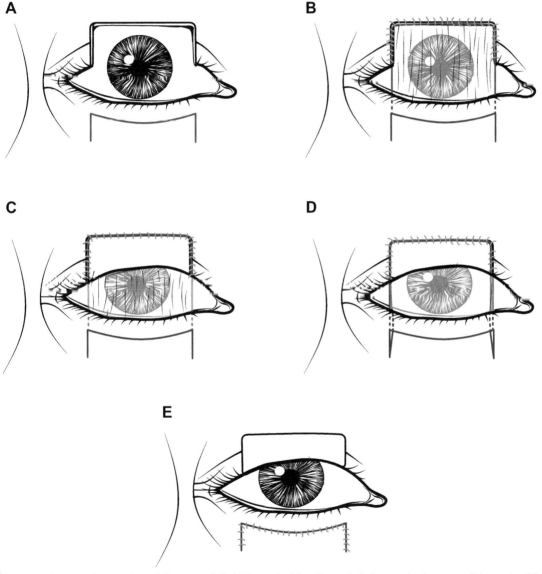

Fig. 6. Cutler-Beard procedure. (A) Create full-thickness incision 5 mm inferior to the lower eyelid margin. (B) Advance the conjunctival flap superiorly and fixate to the upper eyelid conjunctiva and levator aponeurosis. (C) Sew in a posterior lamellar replacement graft to the tarsus and levator aponeurosis. (D) Undermine and then advance the anterior myocutaneous flap into the upper eyelid fixating to skin. (E) Separate the upper and lower eyelids, and inset the lower eyelid tissue.

1. Canthotomy and cantholysis, as described previously. Angle the incision inferiorly to continue as the semicircular flap.
2. Creating the semicircular myocutaneous flap: dissect in a submuscular plane up to the orbital rim and then subcutaneously to avoid branches of the facial nerve (**Fig. 5A**).
3. Anchoring the flap: once the wound edges can be opposed without tension, place a fixation suture, attaching the orbicularis to the periosteum of the lateral orbital rim (**Fig. 5B**).
4. Closing the eyelid margin defect, as described previously.
5. Stabilizing the newly formed eyelid margin with 1 or 2 7-0 Vicryl mattress sutures and reforming the lateral canthal angle by attaching the orbicularis layer to the exposed inferior canthal tendon (**Fig. 5C**).
6. Closing the lateral canthal skin (**Fig. 5D**).

Large Defects

When there is insufficient local upper eyelid tissue to reconstruct the full-thickness defect, distal flaps must be constructed to provide a blood supply for any reconstruction. The classic upper eyelid reconstruction when greater than two-thirds of the eyelid is missing is a Cutler-Beard procedure, which is a 2-stage bridging procedure.[19] The lower eyelid

margin is left intact with inferior full-thickness incision made to advance a skin-muscle conjunctiva into the upper eyelid underneath this bridge of tissue. Modifications to the Cutler-Beard procedure include replacing the tarsal plate to provide stability to the eyelid margin and help prevent entropion.[20] Materials used to replace the rigid posterior lamella are then sandwiched between the conjunctiva and myocutaneous flaps include donor sclera, acellular dermis, and auricular cartilage.[21–23] Mucosa-lined grafts, such as free tarsoconjunctival grafts and hard palate grafts, may be placed at the second stage reconstruction to enforce the margin.[4,24] The flap is then divided 2 to 8 weeks after reconstruction with repair of the lower eyelid donor site and repair of the new eyelid margin to prevent entropion.

The steps of a Cutler-Beard procedure include

1. Creating a full-thickness incision of the lower eyelid 5 mm below the lid margin to avoid devascularization and instability of the lower eyelid margin (**Fig. 6A**).
2. Separating the conjunctival flap from the lower eyelid retractors and dissecting down into the inferior sulcus. Create relaxing incisions and advance into the upper eyelid defect, fixating the superior edge to the levator aponeurosis and conjunctiva (**Fig. 6B**).

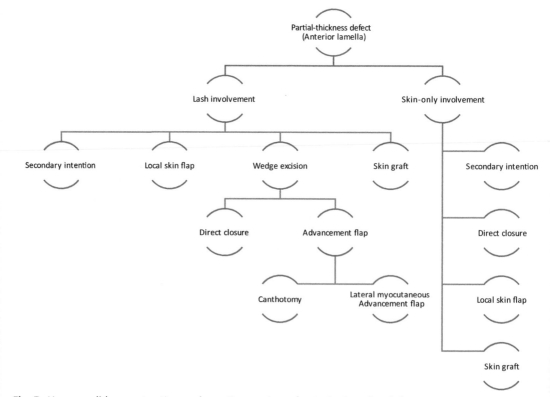

Fig. 7. Upper eyelid reconstruction – schematic overview of anterior lamellar defects.

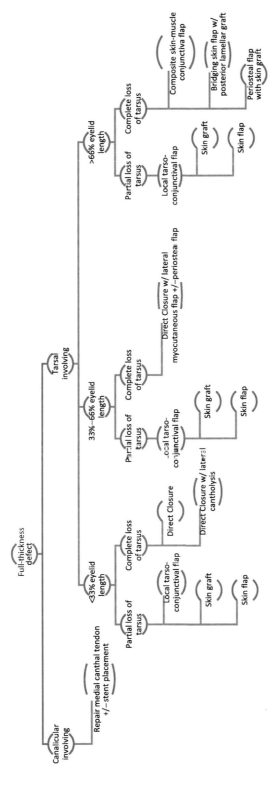

Fig. 8. Upper eyelid reconstruction – schematic overview of full-thickness defects.

3. Sewing in place the posterior lamellar replacement attached to the remaining tarsal edges and the levator aponeurosis (**Fig. 6**C).
4. Dissecting the myocutaneous flap inferiorly as needed down to the orbital rim or into the cheek. Advance the flap under the lower eyelid margin and suture to the upper eyelid tissue (**Fig. 6**D)
5. Separating the upper and lower eyelids; inset the lower eyelid tissue (**Fig. 6**E).

SUMMARY

Reconstruction of eyelid defects requires the integration of many different techniques to achieve the most functional and aesthetic outcome. In a review of outcomes at 6 tertiary oculoplastic centers, Poh and colleagues[25] found that 23% of patients with full-thickness upper eyelid defects required adjunctive surgery, and 56.3% of patients suffered postoperative complications. These included lagophthalmos, exposure keratopathy, upper eyelid retraction, upper eyelid entropion, ptosis, and trichiasis. Being familiar with the most common techniques for repair assists in the complex planning that takes place in the moments after a surgeon is presented with a patient requiring repair, but postoperative care is essential to follow and treat complications that may occur. **Figs. 7** and **8** illustrate a decision tree outlining the options discussed in this review. Facial plastic surgeons should keep in mind that creativity is essential in using these principles with the tissue that is available.

REFERENCES

1. Lowry JC, Bartley GB, Garrity JA. The role of second-intention healing in periocular reconstruction. Ophthal Plast Reconstr Surg 1997;13:174–88.
2. Suryadevara AC, Moe KS. Reconstruction of eyelid defects. Facial Plast Surg Clin North Am 2009;17:419–28.
3. Nerad JA. Oculoplastic surgery. St Louis (MO): Mosby; 2001.
4. Baker SR. Local flaps in facial reconstruction. 2nd edition. Philadelphia: Mosby; 2007.
5. Freitag SK, Lee H, Lee NG, et al. Retrospective review of eyelash number in patients who have undergone full-thickness eyelid resection. Ophthal Plast Reconstr Surg 2014;30:1–6.
6. Rathore DS, Chickadasarahilli S, Crossman R, et al. Full thickness skin grafts in periocular reconstructions: long-term outcomes. Ophthal Plast Reconstr Surg 2014;30:517–20.
7. Bush K, Cartmill BT, Parkin BT. Skin grafts in the periocular region without a bolstered dressing. Orbit 2012;31:59–62.
8. Leibovitch I, Huilgol SC, Richards S, et al. The Australian Mohs database: short-term recipient-site complications in full-thickness skin grafts. Dermatol Surg 2006;32:1364–8.
9. Spinelli HM, Shapiro MD, Wei LL, et al. The role of lacrimal intubation in the management of facial trauma and tumor resection. Plast Reconstr Surg 2005;115:1871–6.
10. Madge SN, Malhotra R, Thaller VT, et al. A systematic approach to the oculoplastic reconstruction of the eyelid medial canthal region after cancer excision. Int Ophthalmol Clin 2009;49:173–94.
11. Howard GR, Nerad JA, Kersten RC. Medial canthoplasty with microplate fixation. Arch Ophthalmol 1992;110:1783–7.
12. Morley AM, deSousa JL, Selva D, et al. Techniques of upper eyelid reconstruction. Surv Ophthalmol 2010;55:256–71.
13. Game J, Morlet N. Lateral canthal fixation using an oblique vertically orientated asymmetric periosteal transposition flap. Clin Experiment Ophthalmol 2007;35:204–7.
14. McCord CD, Boswell CB, Hester TR. Lateral canthal anchoring. Plast Reconstr Surg 2003;112:222–37.
15. Tenzel RR, Stewart WB. Eyelid reconstruction by the semicircle flap technique. Ophthalmology 1978;85:1164–9.
16. Hawes MJ. Free autogenous grafts in eyelid tarsoconjunctival reconstruction. Ophthalmic Surg 1987;18:37–41.
17. Bartley GB, Kay PP. Posterior lamellar eyelid reconstruction with a hard palate mucosal graft. Am J Ophthalmol 1989;107:609–12.
18. Gu J, Zhai J, Chen J. The use of acellular human dermis composite graft for upper eyelid reconstruction in ocular injury. J Trauma Acute Care Surg 2012;72:288–92.
19. Cutler NL, Beard C. A method for partial and total upper lid reconstruction. Am J Ophthalmol 1955;39:1–7.
20. Carrol RP. Entropion following the cutler-beard procedure. Ophthalmology 1983;90:1052–5.
21. Wesley RE, McCord CD. Transplantation of eyebank sclera in the cutler–beard method of upper eyelid reconstruction. Ophthalmology 1980;87:1022–8.
22. Hayek B, Hatef E, Nguyen M, et al. Acellular dermal graft (alloderm) for upper eyelid reconstruction after cancer removal. Ophthal Plast Reconstr Surg 2009;25:426–9.
23. Yaqub A, Leatherbarrow B. The use of autogenous auricular cartilage in the management of upper eyelid entropion. Eye (Lond) 1997;11:801–5.
24. Yoon MK, McCulley TJ. Secondary tarsoconjunctival graft: a modification to the cutler-beard procedure. Ophthal Plast Reconstr Surg 2013;29:227–30.
25. Poh EW, O'Donnell BA, McNab AA, et al. Outcomes of upper eyelid reconstruction. Ophthalmology 2014;121:612–3.e1.

Lower Eyelid Reconstruction

John B. Holds, MD[a,b,c,*]

KEYWORDS

- Lower • Eyelid • Reconstruction • Flap • Graft • Anatomic • Bilayer • Lamella

KEY POINTS

- The eyelid has an anterior lamella of skin and muscle and a posterior lamella of mucosa that must be reconstituted in any reconstruction.
- Composite flaps or an anterior or posterior lamellar flap and opposing graft may be used in reconstruction of the eyelid margin.
- The medial and lateral canthi are vital supportive structures and maintain the shape and position of the eyelid. Their function must be maintained in eyelid reconstruction.
- Whenever possible, the function of the lacrimal canalicular system must be maintained or restored in eyelid reconstruction.
- Surgeons must possess a range of reconstructive options to provide optimal results in eyelid reconstruction.

INTRODUCTION

Knowledge of anatomy and function of the eyelids is essential when faced with the challenges of eyelid reconstruction. Trauma can cause significant tissue loss, which necessitates reconstruction, rather than primary closure, and correcting congenital defects may also require reconstruction and repair. Most commonly, periocular reconstruction follows excision of malignancies. An aesthetically optimal restoration of anatomy and function is always the paramount goal in eyelid reconstruction.

ANATOMY

The eyelids protect and lubricate the ocular surface. The tear film and corneal interface is essential for vision. An inadequate tear film causes blurred vision, infection, and scarring, or even loss, of the eye. With each blink, tears coat the cornea, providing lubrication, essential nutrients, and oxygen to the ocular surface.

The eyelid is made up of anterior and posterior lamellae. The posterior lamella of the eyelid is lined with conjunctiva, a nonkeratinized epithelial mucous membrane filled with secretory glands. Anterior to and intimately attached to the conjunctiva at the lid margin are the more rigid tarsal plates composed of dense connective tissue that provides support to the eyelids. The tarsus has its largest vertical height centrally (10–12 mm upper eyelid and 4 mm lower eyelid) and tapers toward the canthal angles attaching to the canthal tendons.[1]

The anterior lamella consists of the skin and muscle of the eyelid. The skin of the eyelid is unique because it is the thinnest in the body. It is devoid of subcutaneous fat, so the epidermis and dermis directly overlie the orbicularis oculi

[a] Department of Ophthalmology, Saint Louis University School of Medicine, 1755 S. Grand Boulevard, St. Louis, MO 63104, USA; [b] Department of Otolaryngology/Head and Neck Surgery, Saint Louis University School of Medicine, 3635 Vista Avenue, St. Louis, MO 63110, USA; [c] Ophthalmic Plastic and Cosmetic Surgery, Inc., 12990 Manchester Road, #102, Des Peres, MO 63131, USA
* Ophthalmic Plastic and Cosmetic Surgery, Inc., 12990 Manchester Road, #102, Des Peres, MO 63131.
E-mail address: jholds@gmail.com

Facial Plast Surg Clin N Am 24 (2016) 183–191
http://dx.doi.org/10.1016/j.fsc.2016.01.001
1064-7406/16/$ – see front matter © 2016 Elsevier Inc. All rights reserved.

facialplastic.theclinics.com

muscle. The orbicularis oculi is anterior to the tarsal plates and deep to skin. The orbicularis oculi provides for eyelid closure. Forceful closure is obtained from the orbital portion of the muscle, whereas involuntary blink originates from the preseptal and pretarsal portions of the orbicularis oculi. Maintaining orbicularis innervation from the facial nerve is essential to ensure eyelid closure and blink.

The medial and lateral borders of the eyelids are formed by the canthal tendons. The canthal tendons add support to the eyelids and maintain the palpebral fissures. The medial canthal tendon has both anterior and posterior arms that attach to their respective lacrimal crests, encircling the lacrimal sac. Laterally, the canthal tendon attaches above the lateral orbital tubercle, within the orbital rim. The lateral canthal tendon generally attaches 2 mm higher than the medial canthal tendon.[2]

The lacrimal drainage system originates in the eyelids. In the upper and lower eyelids, a punctum is present in the margin, which is the opening to the canaliculi. The first 2 mm of the canaliculi travel vertically from the puncta, before a 90° turn. The canaliculi then run horizontally for 8 mm to 10 mm, beneath skin toward the medial canthal angle. The canaliculi either directly connect to the lacrimal sac or join as a common canaliculus prior to entering the lacrimal sac. The lacrimal sac drains through the nasolacrimal duct beneath the inferior turbinate in the nose.

GENERAL PRINCIPLES OF EYELID RECONSTRUCTION

The end goal of any eyelid reconstruction is an aesthetically optimal restoration of anatomy and anatomic function with a minimum of surgical morbidity. Attention to reconstitution of the bilamellar eyelid structure is essential. The surgeon must create an anterior lamella of adequate and aesthetically appropriate skin, preserving dynamic orbicularis muscle function whenever possible, and create a posterior lamella replacing tarsus at the eyelid margin and providing for a smooth mucosal surface that protects and preserves the cornea.

A preoperative consultation should take place whenever possible so the surgeon can plan an appropriate operative environment and anesthesia and can counsel the patient regarding the probable and extreme possible sizes of the surgical defect and the range of surgical techniques that may have to be used in the repair. Possible sites from which flaps and grafts are to be obtained and the potential for morbidity, the need for temporary eyelid closure, secondary procedures, and risks, such as canalicular obstruction and postoperative tearing, are best explained before tumor resection.

Lower eyelid defects are categorized by amount of full-thickness eyelid defect (as percent of eyelid margin), degree of nonmarginal eyelid involvement, total size of defect, canthal involvement, and lacrimal involvement. Knowledge of an array of reconstructive options allows for planning of the surgical repair.

Many lower eyelid reconstructions are accomplished with a bilamellar advancement of anterior and posterior lamella as a composite flap,[3] most frequently from the lateral canthus.[4] This technique is described in detail later.[5] Defects that require a flap to reconstitute 1 lamella of the eyelid generally use a graft to reconstruct the opposing lamella. It is usually impossible to place a graft on a graft, because there is no blood supply to either graft, and both layers undergo necrosis.[6] The surgeon should consider past or future treatments that may compromise repair, including prior surgery in the area and radiation therapy.

Surgical tension in lower eyelid repair should be directed with tension on flap pedicles directed horizontally, most often superolaterally. Any vertical tension on flaps or vertical recruitment of tissue generally results in retraction of the lower eyelid, which is very hard to correct later.

Appropriate medial and lateral canthal fixation is essential to maintain the position, contour, and horizontal dimension of the eyelid. Direct suturing to periosteum, periosteal flaps,[2] and screw or drill hole fixation are often required to stabilize the position of the reconstructed eyelid and maintain an appropriate eyelid fissure and position.[7] In the medial canthus, the presence of the lacrimal drainage system may necessitate its reconstruction or its sacrifice and later Jones tube (conjunctivodacryocystorhinostomy [CDCR or Jones tube]) surgery.[8]

Nonmarginal eyelid defects can still compromise eyelid function, the position of the eyelid margin, and require careful consideration and reconstruction along the general principles of facial reconstruction.[9–12] Complex defects may extend beyond the surgical skills of a single surgeon and necessitate a multidisciplinary approach to repair.

EYELID DEFECTS AND RECONSTRUCTION

When encountered with full-thickness eyelid defects, replacement of the anterior and posterior lamellae is required for adequate function. Marginal eyelid defects can be classified by the percent of the eyelid margin involved as small (<20%–30%), medium (30%–50%), or large

(>30–50%). A range is applied in this classification to make the point that eyelid laxity, condition of the skin, and prior surgery may convert a small (ie, easily repaired) defect in an older patient with skin and eyelid margin laxity to a medium category defect in a young patient or patient with very tight eyelids, tight skin, or prior surgery.

Table 1 shows a simplified scheme for reconstruction of marginal lower eyelid defects. Familiarity with the limits of each surgical technique allow a surgeon to best choose a reconstructive approach. Special situations that may modify the reconstructive technique include medial and lateral canthal involvement and shallow versus deep defects.

In some instances, such as a marginal laceration or a small vertical defect, the eyelid can be repaired by direct closure. Care should be taken to not simply pull together larger defects in this fashion, as the lateral canthus is pulled medially with rounding and distortion of the eyelid fissure. The goal of this repair is reapproximation of the eyelid, with a continuous lash margin, which provides optimal functional and cosmetic outcome. The technique of marginal eyelid repair is described later.

Defects involving 30% to 50% of the eyelid require advancement and rearrangement of neighboring tissues, sometimes with grafting, to adequately reconstruct the eyelid. The lateral advancement flap is the go-to approach for moderate-sized lower eyelid defects, and it is a basic technique that all surgeons performing eyelid reconstruction must be familiar with.

LATERAL ADVANCEMENT FLAPS

1. The lateral canthal region and eyelid defect are infiltrated with local anesthetic with epinephrine.[5] This repair can be performed under local anesthetic alone or with monitored sedation or general anesthesia.
2. Prepare and drape the surgical sites; place corneal protectors.
3. Mark a lateral canthotomy from the canthal angle 10 mm to 15 mm superior, then lateral from the canthal angle (**Fig. 1**). Make the skin incision with a #15 blade and open through the orbicularis muscle with Westcott scissors.
4. Undermine and release deep to orbicularis, taking care to not disturb the orbicularis muscle and skin of the flap.
5. Perform a cantholysis by strumming the tendon with Westcott scissors for identification, then incising the tendon. Be sure the tendon is fully released to allow advancement of the eyelid (**Fig. 2**).
6. Undermine the flap laterally and inferiorly until there is enough advancement to approximate the tarsus with minimal tension.
7. Using 5-0 or 6-0 Vicryl suture, take partial thickness bites of the tarsal plate, ensuring there is proper alignment (**Fig. 3**). Preplace 2 to 3 bites, and tie all with placement confirmed.
8. Place two 6-0 silk sutures along the eyelid margin to align and approximate the lashes and lid margin. Through the meibomian gland orifices is a good posterior first suture location, with the second aligning the lash follicles. These sutures are tied and the tails left long to tie over inferiorly, preventing the suture tails from irritating the ocular surface (**Fig. 4**).
9. Reform the canthal angle by placing 5-0 or 6-0 Vicryl sutures through the lateral canthal tendon, the periosteum of the orbital rim, and, finally, through the orbicularis muscle of the flap (**Fig. 5**).

Table 1		
Treatment of full-thickness lower eyelid defects		
Full-thickness Defect Size	**Primary Techniques**	**Adjunct Techniques**
Small (20%–30%)	Direct closure	—
	Canthotomy with closure	—
	Lateral advancement flap	—
Medium (30%–40%)	Lateral advancement flap	Canthal fixation
		Canalicular reconstruction
		Periosteal flap
Large (>40–50%)	Lateral advancement flap	—
	Hughes tarsoconjunctival flap	FTSG
	Mustarde cheek flap	Autogenous tarsal graft or hard palate mucosal graft
		Medial canthotomy/cantholysis[21]

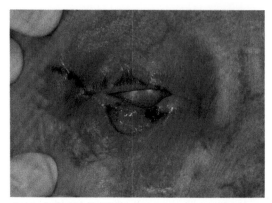

Fig. 1. A 50% full-thickness lower eyelid defect (once tarsal edges are squared) showing superior, then lateral, incision.

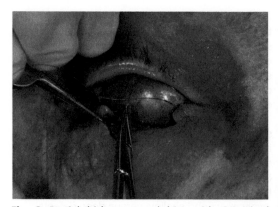

Fig. 3. Partial-thickness tarsal bite with 6-0 Vicryl suture.

10. Once deep sutures are in place, close the skin (**Fig. 6**).
11. Place antibiotic ointment in the eye and incisions.
12. Leave sutures in place for 7 to 12 days.

Eyelid defects larger than 40% to 50% are technically more challenging to repair. The amount of missing posterior lamella in defects this size usually makes lateral advancement alone ineffective. A vascularized flap is created with conjunctiva and tarsus, requiring a 2-stage operation with occlusion of the eye for 3 to 4 weeks.[6,13]

Another alternative for large, full-thickness eyelid defects is a free tarsal graft with an overlying vascularized flap.[14,15] The donor site is the tarsus of the opposite upper eyelid. This is a simple graft to harvest, with the eyelid anesthetized and everted and the tarsus harvested from the upper edge of the tarsus, keeping 2.5 mm to 3 mm of marginal tarsus undisturbed. If there is no good option for a tarsal graft, hard palate mucosa,[16]

nasal chondromucosa, ear cartilage,[17] and commercially available tissue grafts[18] can be substituted.

TARSOCONJUNCTIVAL FLAP (HUGHES FLAP) TO REPAIR A LOWER EYELID DEFECT (STAGE I)

1. Anesthetize the involved upper and lower eyelids along with a donor site for a skin graft with local anesthetic with epinephrine.[6,13] This procedure can be performed under local anesthesia but is easier to perform under monitored sedation or general anesthesia.
2. Prepare and drape the full face including the donor site for the full-thickness skin graft (FTSG).
3. Place a corneal protector and measure the defect size.
4. Evert the upper eyelid and mark a transverse horizontal incision, leaving 2.5 mm to 3 mm of marginal tarsus. Also mark the horizontal

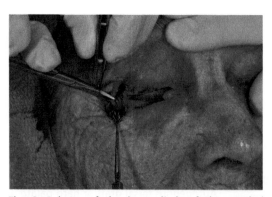

Fig. 2. Release of the lower limb of the canthal tendon leaving the overlying skin and muscle undisturbed.

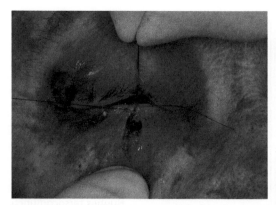

Fig. 4. 6-0 or 7-0 silk sutures are placed in the eyelid margin to approximate the eyelid. The suture ends can be tied over as illustrated, or 7-0 chromic gut sutures can be placed and cut on the knot.

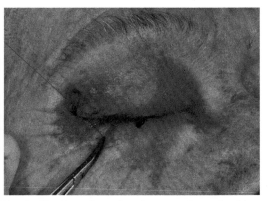

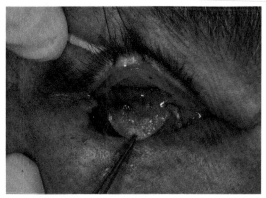

Fig. 5. The lateral canthus is approximated with a buried 5-0 or 6-0 Vicryl suture suturing the lateral upper lid to the periosteum and back through the orbicularis muscle underlying the advancement flap.

Fig. 7. Horizontal, then vertical, tarsal, and conjunctival incisions release the tarsoconjunctival flap to reflect into the eyelid defect.

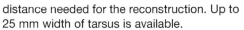

distance needed for the reconstruction. Up to 25 mm width of tarsus is available.

5. Incise horizontally paralleling the eyelid margin. Raise the tarsus making superior conjunctival incisions and reflecting the tarsus inferiorly into the defect (**Fig. 7**).
6. Horizontally divide Muller muscle 3-4 mm above the upper edge of tarsus across the width of the flap, then bluntly recess it 3-4 mm.
7. Remove the corneal protector.
8. Advance the tarsoconjunctival flap and suture to the free ends of the tarsal graft to the remaining lower eyelid tarsal tissue with 6-0 Vicryl (**Fig. 8**).
9. Cover the lower eyelid anterior lamellar defect with either an FTSG or a skin transposition flap (**Fig. 9**).
10. An alternate technique for tarsoconjunctival flap elevation is to leave Müller muscle intact. The flap pedicle is more robust, but opening

the flap is much more difficult, because the scarred Müller muscle plane must be carefully recessed at the time the flap is opened. Failure to adequately recess Müller muscle results in upper eyelid retraction.

TARSOCONJUNCTIVAL FLAP (HUGHES FLAP) TO REPAIR A LOWER EYELID DEFECT (STAGE 2—3 TO 6 WEEKS AFTER INITIAL PLACEMENT)

1. Anesthetize the upper and lower eyelids with local anesthetic with epinephrine. This procedure can be performed with or without monitored sedation.
2. Prepare and drape the surgical site.
3. Using a skin rake, gently elevate the margin of the upper eyelid.
4. Determine the location to separate the lower eyelid tarsoconjunctival graft from the upper eyelid. (Note: in general, separate the tissue

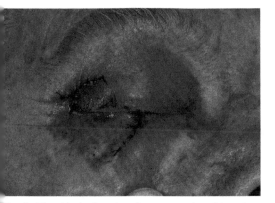

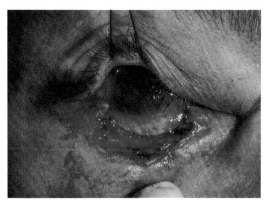

Fig. 6. The skin is closed and rearranged excising dog-ears.

Fig. 8. The tarsoconjunctival flap is released and reflected into the defect, shown after releasing Müller muscle.

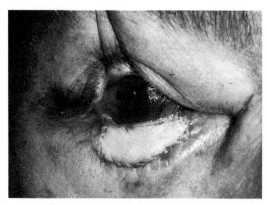

Fig. 9. After placement of the skin graft and prior to placing a bolster. This flap is robust and skin graft failure is rare.

with 1–2 mm override on the lower eyelid, because the graft has a tendency to retract.)
5. Separate the upper and lower eyelids using a scissor.
6. Excise redundant conjunctiva from upper eyelid. Apply bipolar cautery for hemostasis.

CANTHAL DEFECTS AND RECONSTRUCTION

A lid margin laceration or defect extending medial to the puncta, a canalicular laceration, or defect must be suspected. The integrity of the lacrimal system is verified by probing with a Bowman probe. If a laceration or defect is present, canalicular stents are place during eyelid reconstruction.[8] Stents are left in place for 3 to 4 months to ensure complete healing. Failure to repair damage to the lacrimal system results in persistent tearing that is challenging to repair, with more limited options at a later date.

Canalicular Probing and Bicanalicular Intubation

1. Dilate the lacrimal puncta and probe the system using Bowman probes.
2. If a defect is noted, the nose is packed with cottonoid strips soaked in oxymetazoline nasal spray or 4% cocaine beneath the inferior turbinate.
3. A silicone bicanalicular lacrimal stent is placed through the puncta and canaliculus.
4. Inspect the medial canthus to find the stump of the lower canaliculus. Once found, thread the lacrimal stent through the canaliculus into the lacrimal sac and down the nasolacrimal duct. Probe and pass the stent delicately to avoid false passages. If there is difficulty finding the proximal end of the canaliculus, a pigtail probe

can often be carefully placed through the intact canaliculus to act as a guide.
5. Retrieve the stents in the nose, beneath the inferior turbinate. The stent is retrieved with a Crawford hook, groove director, or hemostat.
6. Repair any soft tissue defects of the medial canthus with 5-0 Vicryl sutures. If the suture needle nicks any part of the silicone intubation stents, they tear and require replacement. When placing deep sutures, ensure that the medial canthus is reapproximated back to its posterior location (**Fig. 10**).
7. Remove the metal probes from the silicone stents and tie in a square knot within the nose. Check to ensure there is not tension on the puncta, because the stents can erode through the system if too tight.

When reattaching the medial canthal tendon, care must be taken to ensure that the canalicular system remains intact and that the canalicular stents are not damaged by suture needles. The canthal tendon needs to be reattached back in its posterior position by sutures, wires, or fixation with plates to the nose. If there is loss of the medial canthal tendon, a periosteal flap can be constructed. If there is no tissue loss, the skin and muscle should be reapproximated and closed with deep absorbable sutures (5-0 or 6-0 Vicryl) and the skin sutured.

When there is a complete loss of the canalicular system or reconstruction is not possible, an artificial lacrimal drainage system is created later. Conjunctivodacryocystorhinostomy (Jones tube procedure) is a delayed procedure and is generally performed months to years after the repair of cancer defects.

If a skin defect is present in the medial canthus, reconstruction is necessary. Defects involving

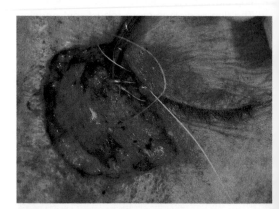

Fig. 10. A large medial canthal defect with upper and lower canalicular defects. The lateral stumps of the eyelid are reimplanted into the medial canthus and the remaining soft tissue defect repaired with flaps and grafts.

both skin and muscle can be repaired by median forehead flaps,[9,11] glabellar flaps,[10] bilobed flaps,[12] island pedicle flaps,[19] and modified rhomboid flaps.[20] Small defects, involving only the skin, are best repaired with an FTSG. Ideal donor sites include excess upper eyelid skin, posterior auricular skin, or skin taken from the medial side of the upper arm. Inspection of donor sites should be done to ensure that there are no lesions being grafted, such as malignancy, and skin should also be inspected to ensure matching of color and texture.

NONMARGINAL EYELID DEFECTS AND RECONSTRUCTION

There are many reconstructive options when closing nonmarginal defects in the periocular area. If the defect involves only the anterior lamella (skin and orbicularis muscle), repairs used elsewhere on the face are appropriate. If a skin defect is present, a skin graft (described previously) or tissue flap can provide an optimal outcome. For larger defects in the anterior lamella, larger flaps, such as the Mustarde cheek flap[13] or rhomboid flaps,[20] provide both functional and cosmetically acceptable outcomes. It is helpful to look at the concept of aesthetic units (eyelid, cheek, and perioral) when designing repairs. For large defects crossing from the eyelid to cheek, it is often appropriate to repair the cheek defect with a flap. If inadequate eyelid skin can be advanced to repair the anterior lamella of the eyelid, a skin graft may provide an optimal match.

Island Pedicle Flap

An island pedicle flap is an ideal reconstructive procedure for many small, circular defects, where there is minimal tissue laxity, especially with defects that cross multiple aesthetic units where the flaps are oriented along the relaxed skin tension lines.

1. Determine the orientation of the island pedicle flap based on tissue laxity (**Fig. 11**).
2. Incise the flap with a #15 blade.
3. Undermine the flaps along the margins, keeping the underlying pedicle intact.
4. Advance the tissue and anchor using deep Vicryl suture in the orbicularis muscle.
5. Close the skin with polypropylene or absorbable sutures (**Figs. 12** and **13**).

POSTOPERATIVE WOUND CARE

Wound care is similar for most periocular procedures. Ophthalmic antibiotic ointment is applied

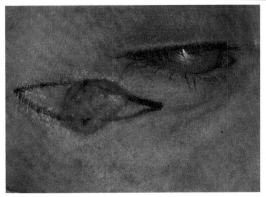

Fig. 11. A moderate-sized defect in a young woman straddling the eyelid-cheek junction. The island pedicles are marked.

2 times per day to the incisions and in the affected eyes at bedtime. Most patients do not tolerate ointment in the eyes throughout the day because it blurs vision. The use of artificial tears 3-6x/day may be needed. Contact lenses cannot be worn while ointment is used during daytime hours.

Current ocular medications, such as glaucoma medications, should be continued throughout the preoperative and postoperative periods. The frequent application of ice packs in the first few postoperative days decreases bruising and swelling. While awake, the patient should be applying ice packs for 20 minutes, with 20-minute intervals between icing.

Sutures are generally removed 6 to 10 days after placement. For skin grafts, I prefer to remove bolsters at 6 to 7 days postoperatively but do not remove the remaining absorbable sutures until 2 to 3 weeks postoperatively. Marginal eyelid defects and other repairs with moderate tension on the wounds have sutures removed closer to 7 to

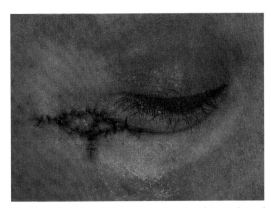

Fig. 12. Island pedicles undermined, advanced, and sutured in place.

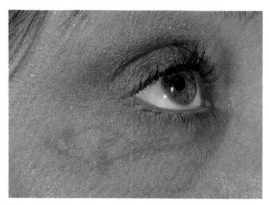

Fig. 13. Patient 3 months postoperatively. Appropriate skin types are present at each level, and the wounds fade with time.

13 days postoperatively. After suture removal, antibiotic ointment is continued for an additional 3 to 7 days.

COMPLICATIONS

After eyelid reconstruction, patients may complain of blurred vision or ocular irritation. This may be secondary to a suture, tissue irritation on the ocular surface, or exposure keratopathy. Decreased orbicularis function may be encountered with lagophthalmos. In addition, swelling can cause mechanical ectropion. Persistent complaints of ocular irritation or vision changes mandate evaluation to ensure that there is no ocular pathology.

Excessive scarring can occur after reconstruction. Hypertrophic scars may be softened with the injection of steroid into the scar (triamcinolone 5 mg/mL). Appropriate scars may be amenable to revision 6 months or more postoperatively. A cicatricial ectropion may occur after reconstructive surgery. These usually result from hypertrophic scarring and skin shortage. I recommend deferring repair for 6 months, if possible, to allow for maturation of the scars. A repair of cicatricial ectropion repair generally involves the release of scar tissue and FTSG.

SUMMARY

An understanding of the anatomy and function of the eyelids is required to provide the best functional and cosmetic outcome for periocular reconstruction. No one reconstructive technique repairs all defects. Knowledge of a range of reconstructive options allows surgeons to offer an optimal surgical plan to patients.

REFERENCES

1. Holds JB, Mohadjer Y. Ch 63 Periocular and lid reconstruction in advanced therapy in facial plastic and reconstructive surgery. In: Regan Thomas J, editor. Shelton (CT): Peoples Medical Publishing House; 2010. p. 735–43.
2. Weinstein GS, Anderson RL, Tse DT, et al. The use of a periosteal strip for eyelid reconstruction. Arch Ophthalmol 1985;103(3):357–9.
3. Anderson RL, Weinstein GS. Full-thickness bi-pedicle flap for total lower eyelid reconstruction. Arch Ophthalmol 1987;105(4):570–6.
4. Tenzel RR, Stewart WB. Eyelid reconstruction by the semicircle flap technique. Ophthalmology 1978;85(11):1164–9.
5. Jordan DR, Anderson RL, Holds JB. Modifications to the semicircular flap technique in eyelid reconstruction. Can J Ophthalmol 1992;27:130–6.
6. Hughes WL. Total lower lid reconstruction: technical details. Trans Am Ophthalmol Soc 1976;74:321–9.
7. Howard GR, Nerad JA, Kersten RC. Medial canthoplasty with microplate fixation. Arch Ophthalmol 1992;110(12):1793–7.
8. Della Rocca DA, Ahmad SM, Della Rocca RC. Direct repair of canalicular lacerations. Facial Plast Surg 2007;23(3):149–55.
9. Field LM. The midline forehead island flap. J Dermatol Surg Oncol 1987;13(3):243–6.
10. Koch CA, Archibald DJ, Friedman O. Glabellar flaps in nasal reconstruction. Facial Plast Surg Clin North Am 2011;19(1):113–22.
11. Sakai S, Soeda S, Matsukawa A. Refinements of the island median forehead flap for reconstruction of the medial canthal area. J Dermatol Surg Oncol 1989;15(5):524–30.
12. Sullivan TJ, Bray LC. The bilobed flap in medial canthal reconstruction. Aust N Z J Ophthalmol 1995;23(1):42–8.
13. Iliff CE, Iliff NT. Partial and total reconstruction of the lower eyelid. Ophthalmology 1980;87(4):272–8.
14. Brown BZ. The use of homologous tarsus as a donor graft in lid surgery. Ophthal Plast Reconstr Surg 1985;1(2):91–5.
15. Stephenson CM, Brown BZ. The use of tarsus as a free autogenous graft in eyelid surgery. Ophthal Plast Reconstr Surg 1985;1(1):43–50.
16. Bartley GB, Kay PP. Posterior lamellar eyelid reconstruction with a hard palate mucosal graft. Am J Ophthalmol 1989;107(6):609–12.
17. Baylis HI, Rosen N, Neuhaus RW. Obtaining auricular cartilage for reconstructive surgery. Am J Ophthalmol 1982;93(6):709–12.
18. Liao SL, Wei YH. Correction of lower lid retraction using tarSys bioengineered grafts for graves ophthalmopathy. Am J Ophthalmol 2013;156(2):387–92.

19. Stephenson C. Reconstruction of the eyelid using a myocutaneous island flap. Ophthalmology 1983; 90(9):1060–5.

20. Teske SA, Kersten RC, Devoto MH, et al. The modified rhomboid transposition flap in periocular reconstruction. Ophthal Plast Reconstr Surg 1998; 14(5):360–6.

21. Holds JB, Anderson RL. Medial canthotomy and cantholysis in eyelid reconstruction. Am J Ophthalmol 1993;116:218–23.

Complications in Eyelid Surgery

Kaveh Karimnejad, MD, Scott Walen, MD, FRCS(C)*

KEYWORDS

- Eyelid • Complications • Blepharoplasty • Eyelid reconstruction • Oculoplastic surgery
- Facial plastic surgery

KEY POINTS

- Preoperative consultation, ophthalmologic/eyelid examination, planning, and meticulous surgical technique are paramount in avoiding postoperative complications after eyelid surgery.
- Counseling the patient about what they can expect in the days to weeks after eyelid surgery is extremely important.
- Complications can range from those that are inherent to any surgery (infection, bleeding, scar) to severe complications that are irreversible (blindness).

INTRODUCTION

The upper and lower eyelids serve functional and cosmetic purposes. Functionally, the eyelids serve to protect the globe from injury. They are also vital to globe protection through the maintenance of tear film, distributing tear film over the cornea, and to regulate the physiologic flow of tear film. The eyelids and periorbital region are central to the perception of facial beauty and aging. The anatomy of the upper and lower eyelids is complex, and altering one structure may have consequences for the entire anatomic unit. A successful surgical procedure preserves the vital function of the eyelid, while maintaining proper symmetry and aesthetic proportions.

Cosmetic blepharoplasty is one of the most common surgical procedures performed in the United States.[1] The main purpose of blepharoplasty is to restore a youthful appearance and bring attention back to the eyes. Eyelid reconstruction, particularly after skin cancer excision, is also common given the high frequency of skin cancer in the general population.[2] Most postoperative eyelid complications are transient and easily

treated (infection, granuloma), whereas there are select complications that can have significant consequences (ptosis, ectropion, irreversible blindness) (**Boxes 1** and **2**). Complications resulting from eyelid surgery are prevented by detailed patient analysis, meticulous surgical technique, and appropriate postoperative care.

PREOPERATIVE HISTORY

Before planning any surgery involving the periorbital region, a thorough patient history must occur (**Box 3**). During this history, it is of upmost importance that patient motivations and expectations are discussed. During the history, the surgeon should look for potential "red flags" that may predispose the patient to complications in the intraoperative or postoperative period (**Box 4**). The patient must provide a detailed list of all medications, including herbals and supplements. The use of anticoagulants and antiplatelet medications is important in that these may cause problematic bleeding, but stopping these medications in the perioperative period is a complex decision and should be done in concert with the patient's

Disclosure Statement: The authors have nothing to disclose.
Department of Otolaryngology-Head and Neck Surgery, Saint Louis University, 3635 Vista Avenue, 6FDT, St Louis, MO 63110, USA
* Corresponding author.
E-mail address: swalen@slu.edu

Facial Plast Surg Clin N Am 24 (2016) 193–203
http://dx.doi.org/10.1016/j.fsc.2015.12.008

Box 1
Functional eyelid complications

- Suture granuloma
- Infection
- Epiphora
- Eyelid hematoma
- Lagophthalmos
- Dry eye syndrome
- Eyelid retraction
- Chemosis
- Diplopia
- Ptosis
- Corneal abrasion/ulcer
- Retrobulbar hematoma
- Blindness

Box 3
History key points

- Patient expectations/motivations
- Ophthalmologic history
- Dry eye symptoms? (burning, foreign body sensation)
- Medications/herbals (anticoagulants/anti-platelet drugs)
- Does the patient use artificial tears?
- Systemic diseases/neuromuscular diseases
- Previous ocular procedures (laser in situ keratomileusis)?
- Previous cosmetic procedures/surgery?
- Relevant scarring history?
- Tobacco use
- Workplace hazards?

primary care physician.[3] In addition, the use of artificial tears regularly or on an as needed basis must be determined because many patients may not consider artificial tears as a medication.

In eyelid surgery, there are specific elements within the medical history that are specifically of concern. A history of other ophthalmologic conditions, dry eye symptoms, previous orbital surgery, systemic diseases, neuromuscular conditions, and scar formation should be discussed before surgery. When discussing ophthalmologic conditions or procedures, a history of laser in situ keratomileusis is important because it may predispose the patient to dry eye symptoms after surgery.[4] Systemic diseases and neuromuscular conditions to be aware of include Graves disease, Sjögren syndrome, rheumatoid arthritis, Bell palsy, and myasthenia gravis. Scar formation is an important topic to address because certain patients, particularly those with darker skin pigmentation, may be predisposed to poor scar or keloid formation.

PERIOCULAR/OCULAR EXAMINATION

A thorough periocular and orbital examination should be performed in any patient undergoing cosmetic or functional procedures of the eyelid (**Box 5**). Ideally, a visual acuity measurement should be undertaken using a standard eye chart. The reactivity of the pupils and ocular motility should also be recorded. A slit-lamp evaluation is a standard examination to rule out any ocular surface irregularities and is a common examination performed by an ophthalmologist. If a surgeon does not routinely perform the previously

Box 2
Cosmetic eyelid complications

- Wound dehiscence
- Suture milia
- Suture granuloma
- Scar/web formation
- Chemosis
- Ptosis
- Deep superior sulcus
- Lower eyelid hollowing
- Eyelid crease asymmetry
- Overcorrection
- Undercorrection

Box 4
"Red flag" patients

- Psychiatric/psychological difficulties
- Recent motivations (job/divorce)
- Unrealistic expectations
- Dry eye symptoms
- Thyroid orbitopathy (Graves disease)
- Anticoagulants/antiplatelet medication
- Lower lid laxity
- Scleral show
- Negative vector eyelid

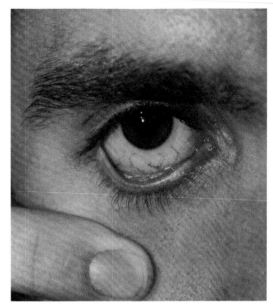

Fig. 1. The snap-test is used to detect the absence of lower eyelid tone. The lower eyelid is displaced inferiorly, toward the orbital rim and then released. A slow return of the lid to normal position reflects poor tone.

mentioned tests, a referral to an ophthalmologist is warranted.

Examining and recording details about the brow and upper eyelid is essential and may help prevent complications including lagophthalmos, ptosis, upper eyelid malposition, and lacrimal gland injury. The height, contour, and position of the brow is important and this should be considered one unit, "the brow-lid continuum." Brow and upper eyelid ptosis should be recorded and explained to the patient, in addition to any preoperative asymmetries that are noticed in the physical examination or photographs. Other important details to record are the position of the upper eye crease and upper eyelid fullness that may be a manifestation of a prolapsed lacrimal gland.

Lower eyelid evaluation is important to avoid classic postoperative complications including chemosis, ectropion, malposition of the lid, and dry eye syndrome (DES). The classic examination maneuver to assess lid laxity is the snap-test, where the examiner's index finger is used to provide downward traction on the lower eyelid and then abruptly released (**Fig. 1**). If the eyelid returns to the globe, this indicates a normal eyelid tone. Another examination maneuver to assess the lower eyelid is the distraction test where the examiner pulls the lower eyelid in an anterior vector. If the eyelid is able to be pulled 6 to 8 mm, this indicates lower lid laxity (**Fig. 2**). The position of the medial and lateral canthus, the lower eyelid-cheek junction, and the presence of a negative vector eyelid should also be assessed. A negative vector eyelid is described as a prominent globe with a retrusive orbital rim (**Fig. 3**).[5] Patients with a negative vector lower eyelid are at an increased complication rate, particularly malposition of the eyelid.

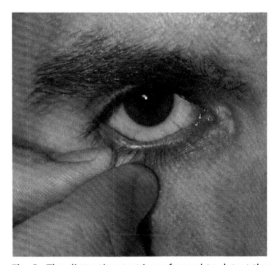

Fig. 2. The distraction test is performed to detect the tone of the lower eyelid. This test is performed by grasping the eyelid gently and pulling anteriorly. If the distance of distraction exceeds 6 to 8 mm, then lower lid laxity is present.

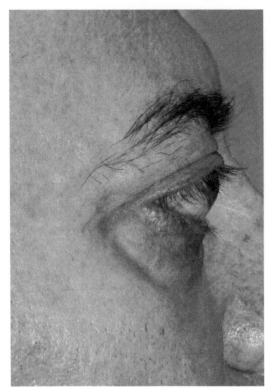

Fig. 3. Lateral view of a patient with a negative vector lower eyelid. In a negative vector eyelid, the globe protrudes past the infraorbital rim. (*Courtesy of* Steven Couch, MD, St Louis, MO.)

COMPLICATIONS
Infection

Infection following blepharoplasty is rare given the high vascularity of the eyelids. Carter and colleagues[6] reported a 0.2% infection rate after blepharoplasty without laser resurfacing and a 0.4% infection rate in those that had laser resurfacing. If a true postblepharoplasty infection does occur, treatment depends on the extent of disease. The most common causative pathogens are normal skin flora, but *Streptococcus* and *Mycobacteria* have also been reported.[7,8] Minor cellulitis is usually successfully treated with a third-generation cephalosporin or fluoroquinolone.

Orbital cellulitis is more severe and manifests as excessive pain, eyelid swelling and erythema, decreased visual acuity, and extraocular muscle immobility.[9] Contrast-enhanced computed tomography is necessary to rule out postseptal infection, abscess formation, or even cavernous sinus thrombosis. *Streptococcus*, *Staphylococcus*, and *Mycobacterium* are the most common offending bacteria that cause orbital cellulitis (**Fig. 4**). These patients are managed with broad-spectrum intravenous antibiotics and,

in cases of abscess formation, surgical drainage. Overall, the infection rate for outpatient eyelid surgery is extremely low. Perioperative prophylactic antibiotic administration is not necessary in routine blepharoplasty because topical antibiotics in the postoperative period are sufficient for infection prevention.[10]

Scarring/Web Formation

Eyelid skin has a tendency to heal well; however, scar formation following blepharoplasty may occur as a result of inadequate surgical technique or in patients with poor physiologic wound healing. Cicatricial medial or lateral canthal webbing is particularly troublesome following blepharoplasty because it can cause aesthetic and functional impairment. Cicatricial canthal webs are semilunar folds of skin with an associated scar, which obscures underlying tissues similar to an epicanthal fold. Functional impairment usually consists of reduced field of vision on lateral gaze.[11]

Risk factors for postoperative medial canthal webbing include a pre-existing tarsal fold and aggressive excision of medial eyelid and nasal skin during surgery. Medial webbing commonly is a result of extending a blepharoplasty too close to the lid margin, angling the incision inferiorly, or too medially. Lateral webbing may be a result of the upper and lower incisions forming an inferior angle or if there is aggressive skin removal (**Fig. 5**). Maintaining a distance of 5 mm between the upper and lower incisions may prevent lateral

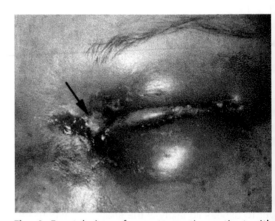

Fig. 4. Frontal view of a postoperative patient with group A, beta-hemolytic streptococcus infection of the right orbit after blepharoplasty. Ruptured violaceous bulla with overlying necrotic tissue in the medial canthal region (*black arrow*). (*From* Goldberg RA, Li TG. Postoperative infection with group A beta-hemolytic *Streptococcus* after blepharoplasty. Am J Ophthalmol 2002;134(6):909; with permission.)

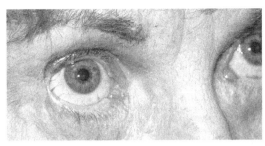

Fig. 5. Oblique view of a patient with significant webbing of the right lateral canthus. The web is particularly accentuated with brow elevation and upgaze. (*From* Lee HB, Bradley EA. Surgical repair of lateral canthal web. Am J Ophthalmol 2006;142(2):339; with permission.)

webbing. Asian patients, patients with brow ptosis, and patients that have a lower eyelid crease may be at a higher risk of webbing in the postoperative period.

Mild canthal webbing may improve with time and gentle massage; however, moderate to severe webbing is a considerable challenge because it often requires a revision surgery that involves complex tissue rearrangement with microflaps. Surgical correction of webbing should be offered after a period of 3 to 6 months after the original procedure. Favored techniques for repair of canthal webbing are Y-V advancement, Z-plasty, or a combination of the two.[12,13]

Eyelid Hematoma

Eyelid hematomas usually present with ecchymosis and mild compressible swelling of the eyelid or peribulbar region. Bleeding typically occurs from the orbicularis muscle or vessels within the orbital fat pads, thus meticulous hemostasis is important for prevention. When patients present with an eyelid hematoma, the first priority is to rule out a retrobulbar hemorrhage (RBH) by evaluating for severe pain or vision changes. Small superficial eyelid hematomas are treated conservatively with head of bed elevation and ice compresses because these usually resolve spontaneously. Larger stable hematomas may be monitored clinically for liquefaction; however, expanding hematomas require immediate surgical exploration, hematoma evacuation, and control of the bleeding source.[9]

Eyelid Crease Asymmetry

Cosmetic and reconstructive surgery of the eyelids may result in a manipulation of the eyelid crease and could result in asymmetry postoperatively.

Often, patient attention is drawn to asymmetries between the eyelids early in the postoperative period. This puts an emphasis on preoperative counseling, and more specifically, analysis of preoperative photographs. Preoperative photography is paramount in surgical planning to obtain a successful result. The patient should also be made aware of asymmetry between their eyes before surgery because this may alter their attitudes and beliefs of the postoperative result (**Fig. 6**).

There are measures that the surgeon can use to minimize further asymmetry postoperatively and this begins when marking the patient preoperatively. Marking the upper eyelid crease and determining the optimal amount of skin excision is one of the most important steps of upper eyelid surgery. If an anatomically correct upper eyelid crease is present, the goal should be to maintain this position. If the upper eyelid crease is absent, or abnormally placed, a general rule is that the crease should be placed 7 to 8 mm above the lash line in white men and 8 to 10 mm above the lash line in white women. Classically, the Asian blepharoplasty results in formation of an upper eyelid crease and this is done by setting the crease between 5 to 6 mm above the lash line in men and 6 to 7 mm in women.

If the upper eyelid creases are asymmetric postoperatively, the surgeon and patient are best advised to wait 3 to 6 months for postoperative swelling to resolve. If the crease is too low on one side, a revision procedure can be performed, which sets the crease higher by making the incision superior to the eyelid crease and fixating orbicularis to the levator aponeurosis at the desired height. If the crease is too high, an incision can be made at the lower level and by using preaponeurotic fat or free fat pearls, readhesion to the higher level can be prevented.

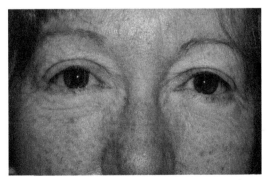

Fig. 6. Frontal view of a preoperative patient with upper eyelid crease asymmetry. (*Courtesy of* Steven Couch, MD, St Louis, MO.)

Lower Eyelid Retraction/Ectropion

Lower eyelid retraction and ectropion are relatively common and problematic complications of lower lid surgery. Retraction is defined as inferior malposition of the lower eyelid margin without eversion. Ectropion is defined as eyelid malposition with lid margin eversion from the globe (**Fig. 7**). When lower eyelid retraction occurs, scleral show, lateral canthal rounding, corneal exposure, and lagophthalmos can occur. This results from inflammation and resultant scarring, followed by vertical shortening of the middle and posterior lamella caused by surgical manipulation.

Ectropion results from excessive skin excision during a transcutaneous blepharoplasty and an unrecognized preoperative lower lid laxity. This can also occur after Mohs surgery resections and reconstructions (**Fig. 8**). Ectropion causes significant postoperative issues including irritation and pain from exposed conjunctiva. Cicatrical ectropion may be avoided by using a transconjunctival blepharoplasty approach, thereby minimizing skin excision and manipulation of the orbital septum and resultant scarring.

Initial treatment of lower lid retraction includes scar massage, artificial tears, and ophthalmic

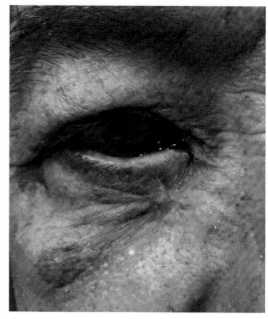

Fig. 8. Frontal view of a patient who underwent Mohs excision and reconstruction with a full-thickness skin graft 3 weeks previous. The patient has lower eyelid retraction and ectropion. This resolved with scar massage and steroid injection.

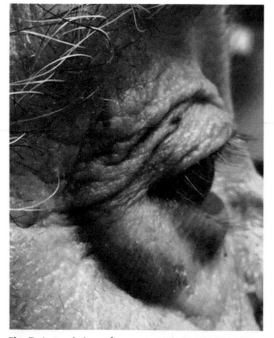

Fig. 7. Lateral view of a preoperative patient with ectropion. This patient also has lower lid retraction. Note that the lower lid margin does not appose the globe.

lubricant. There are a variety of surgical procedures that can address lower lid laxity by anchoring the lateral canthus (canthopexy, canthoplasty, canthal plication, and tarsal strip).[14–32] A transconjunctival approach to the orbital septum, release of scar tissue, and use of a posterior lamellar spacer graft should also be performed for severe lower lid retraction. Ectropion repair may require a spacer graft in the form of a full-thickness skin graft.

Ptosis

Ptosis is a common postoperative finding following blepharoplasty. However, ptosis is not always a sequela of the surgery. Ptosis is often not detected during preoperative evaluation, particularly in patients with extensive dermatochalasis, which can mask the true marginal reflex distance (MRD1), defined as the distance between the center of the pupil in its primary position and the central margin of the upper eyelid. Careful preoperative evaluation should include measurement of MRD1 and palpebral fissure height, and assessment of levator muscle function. If ptosis is discovered preoperatively, operative planning should include ptosis correction at the time of blepharoplasty. Likewise, if levator dehiscence and ptosis is identified intraoperatively, it should be addressed.

Ptosis can occur postoperatively as a result of eyelid edema, ecchymosis, local anesthetic effect, or hematomas.[33] In most of these cases, the effect is temporary. Persistent ptosis may occur as a result of unintended disinsertion of the levator muscle. The levator aponeurosis attaches to orbicularis muscle and skin creating the supratarsal crease; its fibers can be detached during resection of pretarsal orbicularis muscle or preaponeurotic fat. One potential solution is to use a supratarsal fixation suture to reapproximate the aponeurosis to the tarsus.[34] Postoperative ptosis may resolve with time, therefore these patients should be observed for spontaneous recovery for at least 3 months.[35] Finally, surgical correction using levator advancement or Müller muscle resection techniques should be undertaken for unremitting ptosis.[36,37]

Dry Eye Syndrome (Keratoconjunctivitis Sicca)

Dry eyes are a classic and severe complication after eyelid surgery, particularly blepharoplasty. Dry eye symptoms are common in the general population, affecting up to 17% of women and 12% of men. In the literature, there are varying incidences of DES after blepharoplasty, with a range between 8% and 21%.[38–41] In a review of 892 upper and lower blepharoplasties, 26.5% of patients reported dry eye symptoms in the postoperative period. The variables that increase the incidence of DES included male sex, concurrent upper and lower blepharoplasty performed in the same setting, preoperative DES, preoperative skin laxity, hormone therapy, and transcutaneous approaches to the lower eyelid.[42] Other high-risk patients include those with proptosis, lower lid laxity, maxillary hypoplasia, scleral show, and lagophthalmia.

Patients with dry eye symptoms complain of a deep eye pain and discomfort, burning, stinging, foreign-body sensation, blurry vision, photophobia, general orbital irritation, and redness. On physical examination, the conjunctiva appears irritated and red. In the preoperative period, the Schirmer test may be used to assess possible DES. This examination involves placing a Schirmer strip into the lower limbus after a topical anesthetic has been placed into the eye (**Fig. 9**). After 5 minutes, the strip is removed from the limbus and the amount of wetting on the strip is measured, normal measurements are between 10 and 15 mm. A measurement less than 5 mm is suggestive of DES.

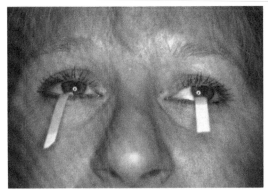

Fig. 9. Patient undergoing the Schirmer test for dry eye syndrome. A strip is inserted into the lateral limbus. After 5 minutes, the strip is removed and the degree of wetting (in millimeters) is measured. Normal range is 10 to 15 mm. If the measurement is less than 10 mm, there is evidence of hyposecretion of tears. (From Meiners PM, Meijer JM, Vissink A, et al. Management of Sjögren's syndrome. In: Weisman MH, Weinblatt ME, Louie JS, et al, editors. Targeted treatment of the rheumatic diseases. Philadelphia: Elsevier; p. 138; with permission.)

The best treatment to avoid dry eye symptoms in the postoperative period is to detect those high-risk patients before surgery. If a patient complains of dry eye symptoms postoperatively, artificial tears and a lubricant can be used to provide comfort and protection to the cornea. Further measures include wearing a patch at night, taping the eye closed, or using a protective corneal lens. Finally, tears may be prevented from draining through the lacrimal system as quickly as by placing punctal plugs, which are made of silicone or hydrogel.

Epiphora

Epiphora is a common complication of lower lid blepharoplasty, particularly in the first few days postoperatively. There are three mechanisms responsible for normal tear production: (1) the production and release of tears from the lacrimal and accessory glands, (2) blinking and distribution of tears, and (3) tear pumping into the lacrimal drainage system.[43] The three most common causes of postblepharoplasty epiphora are corneal irritation, conjunctival chemosis, and lower lid ectropion.[44] Epiphora usually resolves within the first several days postoperatively, particularly if caused by corneal irritation or chemosis. However, if it persists, further evaluation for punctal malpositioning or cannalicular damage should be initiated. Surgical approaches to correct punctal malpositioning include a horizontal tightening procedure, medial spindle procedure, or medial/lateral canthopexy.

Chemosis

Chemosis is defined as transudative edema of the conjunctiva. There are several general causes of chemosis that could be attributable to infection, allergy, or surgery. There are several causes of chemosis in the postoperative patient including exposure of the conjunctiva, periorbital edema, and lymphatic disruption (**Fig. 10**). Chemosis has also been described after canthal disruption during lower lid blepharoplasty. One study looked at 312 primary transcutaneous lower blepharoplasty procedures and found 11.5% incidence of chemosis. Five percent of those patients presented intraoperatively, whereas the remainder of the patients presented over the first postoperative week.[45]

Chemosis presents with edematous and infected conjunctiva (**Fig. 11**). The inflamed tissue may have a clear, yellow, or reddish hue around the cornea. Intraoperatively this can occur because of exposure, which results from lagophthalmos and lack of blink reflex. In the postoperative period, the exposure of the conjunctiva is caused by lagophthalmos. Edema causes chemosis due to the complex lymphatic drainage of the orbit. Finally, natural disruption of lymphatic channels, specifically in lower lid blepharoplasty, leads to lymphatic disruption and chemosis.

Treatment of chemosis starts with prevention intraoperatively using meticulous surgical technique. In the postoperative period, the use of artificial tears during the daytime and ophthalmic lubricant at night for 1 week can help prevent chemosis. If the chemosis is persistent after 1 week, ocular decongestants and ophthalmic steroid drops may be used. Chemosis that continues may also be treated with patching, which provides

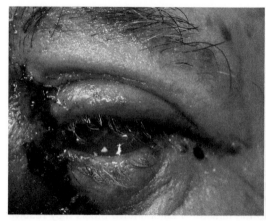

Fig. 11. Left eyelid chemosis after medial canthal tumor removal, including medial conjunctiva, and subsequent repair with a forehead flap.

pressure to the eye. Surgical treatment includes a conjunctivotomy with possible tarsorrhaphy. If the chemosis is caused by lid malposition, this does not resolve until the lid position is corrected. Most cases of chemosis recover spontaneously, or with minimal treatment. Rare cases may last 2 to 6 months and require consistent surveillance and attention to prevent further complications.

Diplopia

Diplopia is a rare but serious complication of blepharoplasty that has been well described in the literature. Transient diplopia may be the result of hematomas, extraocular muscle contracture, wound-related inflammation, or conjunctival edema.[46,47] Edema and hemorrhage in the tissues surrounding the extraocular muscles create a compartment-like syndrome by causing neuromuscular compression and ischemia resulting in extraocular muscle paresis.[48,49] In rare circumstances, diplopia is permanent because of intraoperative structural damage to extraocular muscles causing strabismus, which is a misalignment of the eyes. Extraocular muscle damage is typically the result of overzealous fat excision, deep cautery, or aggressive dissection. The inferior oblique muscle is the most vulnerable to injury given its anatomic location between the medial and central fat compartments and because of its transverse orientation.[50] The inferior oblique can thus be injured during dissection or cauterization of the orbital fat pads and should be carefully identified and protected during fat excision or repositioning. If diplopia persists, the patient should be referred to an ophthalmologist because surgical exploration and strabismus surgery may be warranted.

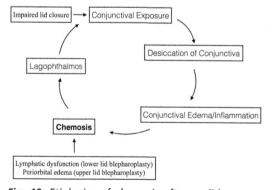

Fig. 10. Etiologies of chemosis after eyelid surgery. This diagram shows the cycle of exposure, dessication, and edema that can occur during and after surgery of the eyelids.

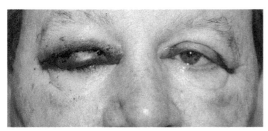

Fig. 12. Right orbital hematoma following bilateral upper eyelid surgery. (*Courtesy of* Steven Couch, MD, St Louis, MO.)

Retrobulbar Hemorrhage

Blindness is the most devastating and most feared complication of blepharoplasty. The most common cause of visual loss following blepharoplasty is RBH. Other less common causes include direct optic nerve injury, central retinal artery occlusion, acute narrow angle glaucoma, and globe perforation. Although the cause of vision loss following RBH is unclear, persistent orbital bleeding causes increased intraorbital pressure with resultant ischemic damage to the optic nerve.[9] The incidence of RBH following blepharoplasty has been reported as 0.05% (1 per 2000) with 0.0045% (1 per 10,000) of patients developing permanent vision loss.[51]

Prevention starts with a thorough preoperative evaluation. Patient risk factors associated with RBH following blepharoplasty include hypertension, antiplatelet and anticoagulant medications, and history of bleeding diathesis or vascular disease. Hypertension is the most common preoperative comorbidity, present in up to 36% of affected patients and must be well controlled before surgery.[51,52] Medications with antiplatelet or anticoagulation properties, such as warfarin, aspirin, or nonsteroidal anti-inflammatory drugs, should be stopped 2 weeks before surgery and for 1 week postoperatively.[52] Herbal supplements with blood thinning properties, such as vitamin E and garlic, should also not be overlooked.[43]

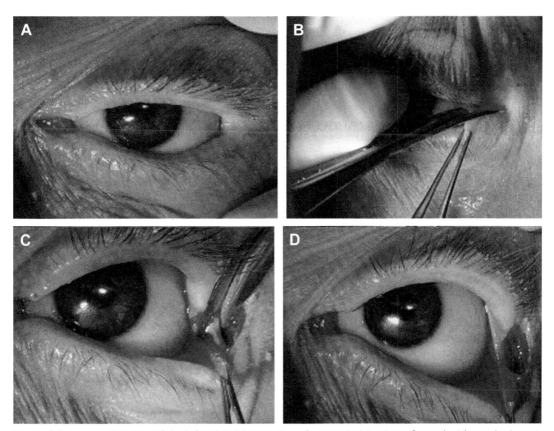

Fig. 13. (*A*) Preoperative view of the left orbit. (*B*) Lateral canthotomy incision is performed with a scalpel or scissors. (*C*) Identification and incision of the inferior canthal tendon, cantholysis. (*D*) Lower eyelid laxity, which allows decompression by allowing the globe and orbital contents to move anterior. (*From* Ramakrishnan VR, Palmer JN. Prevention and management of orbital hematoma. Otolaryngol Clin North Am 2010;43(4):796; with permission.)

There are several intraoperative measures that the surgeon can use to decrease the risk of RBH. Communication with the anesthesiologist to optimize blood pressure control throughout the procedure should occur. The surgeon should wait 10 to 15 minutes following infiltration of local anesthetics with epinephrine to maximize vasoconstriction. Bleeding typically occurs from the orbicularis or vessels within the orbital fat pads, thus meticulous hemostasis is critical before closure and avoidance of excessive traction during fat excision or repositioning. Postoperatively, bleeding is minimized by preventing straining associated with vomiting and coughing by prescribing antitussive and antiemetic medications.

If RBH does occur, most patients (82%) develop signs or symptoms within the first 24 hours with two peaks of presentation, 26% declare intraoperatively or within 1 hour, and 36% declare between 6 and 12 hours postoperatively.[52] The most common symptoms are eye pain and pressure, whereas other signs of RBH include subconjunctival hemorrhage, decreased visual acuity, proptosis, increased intraocular pressure, and an afferent pupillary defect (**Fig. 12**). RBH constitutes an emergency and the surgical incision should be opened immediately for hematoma evacuation. The surgeon should then proceed with lateral canthotomy and cantholysis (**Fig. 13**). If these measures are delayed, the patient may have irreparable damage to vision or ocular motility. Adjunctive therapy to decrease intraocular pressure may include administration of mannitol, dexamethasone, and timolol ophthalmic solution.[53]

SUMMARY

Complications are inevitable in any surgical procedure, despite surgeon talent and preparation. Eyelid surgery, functional and cosmetic, is challenging and mitigating the risks before surgery, meticulous surgical dissection and hemostasis, and ample postoperative care can help minimize the chances of complications. Eyelid complications are functional or cosmetic, but many fall into both categories. Ample communication with the patient about their expectations, their motivations, in addition to educating the patient about potential complications may make for a smoother postoperative course. Recognizing and managing the myriad of potential complications limits the functional and cosmetic morbidity and helps prevent suboptimal results.

REFERENCES

1. International Communications Research. 2011 AAFPRS Membership Study. January 2012:1–35.
2. Medical expenditure panel survey. Rockville (MD): Agency for Healthcare Research and Quality. Available at: http://meps.ahrq.gov/mepsweb/data_stats/download_data_files.jsp. Accessed January 20, 2014.
3. Esparas ES, Sobel RK. Perioperative management of anticoagulants and antiplatelet agents in oculoplastic surgery. Curr Opin Ophthalmol 2015;26(5):422–9.
4. Korn BS, Kikkawa DO, Schanzlin DJ. Blepharoplasty in the post-laser in situ keratomilleusis patient: preoperative considerations to avoid dry eye syndrome. Plast Reconstr Surg 2007;119(7):2232–9.
5. Hirmand H, Codner MA, McCord CD, et al. Prominent eye: operative management of lower lid and midfacial rejuvenation and the morphologic classification system. Plast Reconstr Surg 2002;110:620.
6. Carter SR, Stewart JM, Khan J, et al. Infection after blepharoplasty with and without carbon dioxide laser resurfacing. Ophthalmology 2003;110(7):1430–2.
7. Baudouin C, Pisella PJ, Fillacier K, et al. Ocular surface inflammatory changes induced by topical antiglaucoma drugs: human and animal studies. Ophthalmology 1999;106(3):556–63.
8. Gehrig KA, Warshaw EM. Allergic contact dermatitis to topical antibiotics: epidemiology, responsible allergens, and management. J Am Acad Dermatol 2008;58(1):1–21.
9. Lelli GJ Jr, Lisman RD. Blepharoplasty complications. Plast Reconstr Surg 2010;125(3):1007–17.
10. Lee EW, Holtebeck AC, Harrison AR. Infection rates in outpatient eyelid surgery. Ophthal Plast Reconstr Surg 2009;25(2):109–10.
11. Massry GG. Cicatricial canthal webs. Ophthal Plast Reconstr Surg 2011;27(6):426–30.
12. Field LM. Repair of a cicatricial epicanthal fold by a double Z-plasty (Spaeth). J Dermatol Surg Oncol 1982;8(3):215–7.
13. Lee HB, Bradley EA. Surgical repair of lateral canthal web. Am J Ophthalmol 2006;142(2):339–40.
14. Tenzel RR, Buffman FV, Miller G. The use of the "lateral canthal sling" ectropion repair. Can J Ophthalmol 1977;12:199.
15. Schaefer AJ. Lateral canthal tendon tuck. Am J Ophthalmol 1979;86:1879.
16. Codner MA, McCord CD, Heste TR. The lateral canthoplasty. Oper Tech Plast Reconstr Surg 1998;5:90–8.
17. McCord CD, Codner MA, Hester TR. Redraping the inferior orbicularis arc. Plast Reconstr Surg 1998;102:2471.
18. Flowers RS. Canthopexy as a routine blepharoplasty component. Clin Plast Surg 1993;20:351–65.
19. Lowery JC, Bartley G. Complications of blepharoplasty. Surv Ophthalmol 1983;90:1039–46.

20. Fagien S. Algorithm for canthoplasty: the lateral retinacular suspension: a simplified suture canthopexy. Plast Reconstr Surg 1999;103:2042–53.

21. Jelks GW, Jelks EB. Repair of the lower lid deformities. Clin Plast Surg 1993;20:417.

22. Glat PM, Jelks GW, Jelks EB, et al. Evolution of the lateral canthoplasty: techniques and indications. Plast Reconstr Surg 1997;100:1396.

23. Jelks GW, Glat PM, Jelks EB, et al. The inferior retinacular lateral canthoplasty: a new technique. Plast Reconstr Surg 1997;100:1262.

24. Marsh JL, Edgerton MT. Periosteal pennant lateral canthoplasty. Plast Reconstr Surg 1979;64:24.

25. Patipa M. Lateral canthal tendon resection with conjunctiva preservation for the treatment of lower eyelid laxity during lower eyelid blepharoplasty. Plast Reconstr Surg 1993;91:456.

26. Patipa M. The evaluation and management of lower eyelid retraction following cosmetic surgery. Plast Reconstr Surg 2000;106:438–53.

27. Millman AL, Williams JD, Romo T, et al. The septo-myocutaneous flap in lower lid blepharoplasty. Ophthal Plast Reconstr Surg 1997;13:2–6.

28. McCord CD, Shorr JW. Avoidance of complications in lower-lid blepharoplasty. Ophthalmology 1983; 90:1039–46.

29. Hinderer UT. Correction of weakness of the lower eyelid and lateral canthus. Clin Plast Surg 1993;20:331.

30. Anderson RL, Gordy DD. The tarsal strip procedure. Arch Ophthalmol 1979;97:2192.

31. Pak J, Putterman AM. Revisional eyelid surgery: treatment of severe postblepharoplasty lower eyelid retraction. Facial Plast Surg Clin North Am 2005; 13(4):461–9.

32. Lee AS, Thomas JR. Lower lid blepharoplasty and canthal surgery. Facial Plast Surg Clin North Am 2005;13(4):541–51.

33. Klapper SR, Patrinely JR. Management of cosmetic eyelid surgery complications. Semin Plast Surg 2007;21(1):80–93.

34. McCord CD, Seify H, Codner MA. Transblepharoplasty ptosis repair: three-step technique. Plast Reconstr Surg 2007;120(4):1037–44.

35. Hornblass A. Ptosis and pseudoptosis and blepharoplasty. Clin Plast Surg 1981;8(4):811–30.

36. Carraway JH, Vincent MP. Levator advancement technique for eyelid ptosis. Plast Reconstr Surg 1986;77(3):394–403.

37. Putterman AM, Urist MJ. Muller muscle-conjunctiva resection. Technique for treatment of blepharoptosis. Arch Ophthalmol 1975;93(8):619–23.

38. Floegel I, Horwath-Winter J, Muellner K, et al. A conservative blepharoplasty may be a means of alleviating dry eye symptoms. Acta Ophthalmol Scand 2003;81:230.

39. Hamawy AH, Farkas JP, Fagien S, et al. Preventing and managing dry eyes after periorbital surgery: a retrospective review. Plast Reconstr Surg 2009; 123(1):353–9.

40. Vold SD, Carroll RP, Nelson JD. Dermatochalasis and dry eye. Am J Ophthalmol 1993;115:216.

41. Moss SE, Klein R, Klein BE. Prevalence of and risk factors for dry eye syndrome. Arch Ophthalmol 2000;118:1264–8.

42. Prishmann J, Sufyan A, Ruffin C, et al. Dry eye symptoms and chemosis following blepharoplasty: a 10-year retrospective review of 892 cases in a single-surgeon series. JAMA Facial Plast Surg 2013;15(1): 39–46.

43. Mack WP. Blepharoplasty complications. Facial Plast Surg 2012;28(3):273–87.

44. Leatherbarrow B, Saha K. Complications of blepharoplasty. Facial Plast Surg 2013;29(4):281–8.

45. Weinfeld AB, Burke R, Codner MA. The comprehensive management of chemosis following cosmetic lower blepharoplasty. Plast Reconstr Surg 2008; 122(2):579–86.

46. Galli M. Diplopia following cosmetic surgery. Am Orthopt J 2012;62:19–21.

47. Glavas IP. The diagnosis and management of blepharoplasty complications. Otolaryngol Clin North Am 2005;38(5):1009–21.

48. Smith B, Lisman RD, Simonton J, et al. Volkmann's contracture of the extraocular muscles following blowout fracture. Plast Reconstr Surg 1984;74(2): 200–16.

49. Hayworth RS, Lisman RD, Muchnick RS, et al. Diplopia following blepharoplasty. Ann Ophthalmol 1984;16(5):448–51.

50. Harley RD, Nelson LB, Flanagan JC, et al. Ocular motility disturbances following cosmetic blepharoplasty. Arch Ophthalmol 1986;104(4):542–4.

51. Hass AN, Penne RB, Stefanyszyn MA, et al. Incidence of postblepharoplasty orbital hemorrhage and associated visual loss. Ophthal Plast Reconstr Surg 2004;20(6):426–32.

52. Mejia JD, Egro FM, Nahai F. Visual loss after blepharoplasty: incidence, management, and preventive measures. Aesthet Surg J 2011;31(1):21–9.

53. Terella AM, Wang TD, Kim MM. Complications in periorbital surgery. Facial Plast Surg 2013;29(1): 64–70.

Index

Note: Page numbers of article titles are in **boldface** type.

Facial Plast Surg Clin N Am 24 (2016) 205–217
http://dx.doi.org/10.1016/S1064-7406(16)30009-8

Moving?

Make sure your subscription moves with you!

To notify us of your new address, find your **Clinics Account Number** (located on your mailing label above your name), and contact customer service at:

Email: journalscustomerservice-usa@elsevier.com

800-654-2452 (subscribers in the U.S. & Canada)
314-447-8871 (subscribers outside of the U.S. & Canada)

Fax number: 314-447-8029

Elsevier Health Sciences Division
Subscription Customer Service
3251 Riverport Lane
Maryland Heights, MO 63043

*To ensure uninterrupted delivery of your subscription, please notify us at least 4 weeks in advance of move.